Lab Manual to Accompany

BIOLOGY
of Women

Lab Manual to Accompany

BIOLOGY
of Women

FIFTH EDITION

THERESA M. HORNSTEIN
Lake Superior College
Duluth, MN

JERI SCHWERIN
Lake Superior College
Duluth, MN

DELMAR
CENGAGE Learning·

Australia · Brazil · Japan · Korea · Mexico · Singapore · Spain · United Kingdom · United States

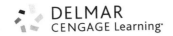

Lab Manual to Accompany Biology of Women, 5th Edition
Theresa M. Hornstein, Jeri Schwerin

Vice President, Editorial: Dave Garza

Executive Editor: Steven Helba

Senior Acquisitions Editor: Maureen Rosener

Managing Editor: Marah Bellegarde

Senior Product Manager: Juliet Steiner

Editorial Assistant: Samantha Miller

Vice President, Marketing: Jennifer Baker

Marketing Director: Wendy Mapstone

Senior Marketing Manager: Michele McTighe

Marketing Coordinator: Scott Chrysler

Production Director: Wendy Troeger

Production Manager: Andrew Crouth

Content Project Manager: Allyson Bozeth

Senior Art Director: Jack Pendleton

For product information and technology assistance, contact us at
Cengage Learning Customer & Sales Support, 1-800-354-9706
For permission to use material from this text or product,
submit all requests online at **www.cengage.com/permissions**.
Further permissions questions can be e-mailed to
permissionrequest@cengage.com

Example: Microsoft ® is a registered trademark of the Microsoft Corporation.

Library of Congress Control Number: 2011934073

ISBN-13: 978-1-4354-0035-1

Delmar
5 Maxwell Drive
Clifton Park, NY 12065-2919
USA

Cengage Learning is a leading provider of customized learning solutions with office locations around the globe, including Singapore, the United Kingdom, Australia, Mexico, Brazil, and Japan. Locate your local office at: **international.cengage.com/region**

Cengage Learning products are represented in Canada by Nelson Education, Ltd.

To learn more about Delmar, visit **www.cengage.com/delmar**

Purchase any of our products at your local college store or at our preferred online store **www.cengagebrain.com**

Notice to the Reader
Publisher does not warrant or guarantee any of the products described herein or perform any independent analysis in connection with any of the product information contained herein. Publisher does not assume, and expressly disclaims, any obligation to obtain and include information other than that provided to it by the manufacturer. The reader is expressly warned to consider and adopt all safety precautions that might be indicated by the activities described herein and to avoid all potential hazards. By following the instructions contained herein, the reader willingly assumes all risks in connection with such instructions. The publisher makes no representations or warranties of any kind, including but not limited to, the warranties of fitness for particular purpose or merchantability, nor are any such representations implied with respect to the material set forth herein, and the publisher takes no responsibility with respect to such material. The publisher shall not be liable for any special, consequential, or exemplary damages resulting, in whole or part, from the readers' use of, or reliance upon, this material.

Printed in the United States of America
1 2 3 4 5 6 7 14 13 12 11

contents

lab exercise 4   ANATOMY OF THE HUMAN
                    BODY—A SYSTEM OVERVIEW   25

lab exercise 5   SKELETAL SYSTEM—DIFFERENCES BETWEEN WOMEN
                    AND MEN   35

lab exercise 6   BLOOD   43

lab exercise 7   FEMALE REPRODUCTIVE SYSTEM   51

lab exercise 8   FEMALE REPRODUCTIVE ANATOMY UNDER
THE MICROSCOPE   59

lab exercise 9   BREAST HEALTH   67

lab exercise 10   HEALTH AND WELLNESS PLANNER   74

lab exercise 11   FITNESS LAB—MEASURING YOUR FITNESS LEVEL   80

lab exercise 16 BIOLOGY OF APPEARANCE   **114**

lab exercise 17 COSMETICS LAB   121

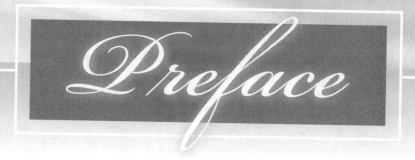

Preface

This lab manual provides students with hands-on experiences designed to complement the material presented in the *Biology of Women* 5th edition. The lab exercises are accessible to entry level students, but offer enough detail and critical thinking opportunities to challenge students who already have some experience in a biology laboratory.

CONCEPTUAL APPROACH

In its position statements, the National Science Teachers Association states:

"At the college level, all students should have opportunities to experience inquiry-based science laboratory investigations . . . . All introductory courses should include labs as an integral part of the science curriculum."
(http://www.nsta.org/about/positions/laboratory.aspx)

Educational research indicates that when students engage in active learning they improve retention and increase understanding. This lab manual offers students opportunities to explore and reinforce their understanding of concepts related to women's biology.

ORGANIZATION OF THE TEXT

A valuable companion to the core book, this student resource provides 17 lab exercises that coordinate with and reinforce the text. The labs are arranged in four units: Introduction to the Lab, Anatomy and Physiology, Fitness and Wellbeing, and Specific Concerns in Women's Health. Covering topics ranging from lab safety and the scientific method, to skeletal system differences between women and men, and a sexually transmitted infections lab, this resource provides everything needed for a successful lab experience.

FEATURES

Within each lab exercise, objectives and materials are outlined, followed by explanations and activities for students to participate in. Each lab exercise concludes with a laboratory report form that includes multiple choice, matching, and long answer response questions.

ALSO AVAILABLE

Biology of Women 5th Edition

ISBN 10: 1-4354-0033-X

ISBN 13: 978-14354-0033-7

Centered on the health of the human female throughout her lifespan, BIOLOGY OF WOMEN, 5th Edition continues to provide an excellent framework to discuss women's physiology, biology, and overall health. Thorough revisions to this benchmark text make the Fifth Edition both scientifically rigorous and socially relevant for today's students.

ABOUT THE AUTHORS

Theresa Hornstein earned an AS from Muskegon Community College, a B.S from Michigan Technological University, and an M.S from the University of Wisconsin Superior. After several years working in labs and field research positions, she moved into teaching both online and in a traditional classroom in the Biology Department at Lake Superior College in Duluth, MN. Courses she has taught include cell biology, microbiology, general biology, botany, science skills, pathophysiology, anatomy and physiology, student research, and biology of women. In addition, she has taught a number of workshops for GirlTech, a local program designed to get 10-14 year old girls interested in science. She has been awarded four Awards for Excellence grants through the Minnesota State Colleges and Universities, as well as serving on the state-wide Task Force for Thinking Assessments and as Center for Teaching and Learning coordinator at Lake Superior College. In 1992, the Minnesota State Board for Community Colleges named her an Outstanding Faculty Member. Her research interests include vermicomposting projects on campus, comparisons of online and on ground student success, applications of the FIRE critical thinking model, edible landscaping, and natural dye projects. She has presented at both regional and national conferences including Fusion2010, I-Teach, the National Science Teachers Association, NISOD, and Women's Lives, Women's Voices, Women's Solutions: Shaping a National Agenda for Women in Higher Education.

Jeri Schwerin earned a B.S. in biology at the University of Minnesota, Duluth; and an M.S. in biology from the University of Massachusetts, Amherst. As a graduate student, she served as a National Science Foundation Teaching Fellow at Hampshire College in Hadley, Massachusetts, and as a program coordinator at the Sigurd Olson Environmental Institute at Northland College in Ashland, Wisconsin. She currently holds a position as a biology instructor at Lake Superior College in Duluth, Minnesota, where she teaches anatomy and physiology, biology and society, and biology of women. In addition to teaching, she serves on the college's Academic Affairs and Standards Council and on the Environmental Council. She has been awarded seven Awards for Excellence by the office of the Chancellor of the Minnesota State Colleges and Universities. In addition to teaching, she currently provides public outreach education with the Lake Superior Research Institute of the University of Wisconsin, Superior on board their research vessel, the LL Smith Jr.

ACKNOWLEDGEMENTS

Jeri Schwerin would like to acknowledge Ellen Kamil, for her encouragement and enduring influence on her life, and on the lives of other women in biology.

Theresa Hornstein would like to thank all the students whose input has helped to refine these labs.

AVENUE FOR FEEDBACK

For comments, questions, or suggestions, please feel free to contact:

Theresa Hornstein   t.hornstein@lsc.edu

Jeri Schwerin   j.schwerin@lsc.edu

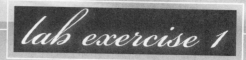

LABORATORY SAFETY

OBJECTIVES

At the completion of this exercise, the student should be able to:

- Identify safety equipment in the lab
- Identify the location of the first aid kit
- Follow the safety procedures for the lab
- Identify lab equipment and the locations of equipment in the lab

MATERIALS

paper and pencil

INTRODUCTION

Most of the laboratory exercises included in the manual do not require direct exposure to chemicals, equipment or body fluids, but some do. Students who are working in a science lab must be aware of the steps they should take to keep themselves and their fellow students safe. It is important to understand how to work safely in the science lab. The following safety precautions have been compiled from information provided by the Centers for Disease Control (CDC). Individual educational institutions may enforce additional precautions or safety rules in their science laboratories.

General Safety Precautions for the Science Laboratory

1. Familiarize yourself with the location of all safety equipment in the laboratory, and with how to operate the equipment. Locate and familiarize yourself with the contents of the first aid kit.

2. Counter and table surfaces in science laboratories can have residues that are toxic if ingested. Do not eat, drink, smoke or store food in the science laboratory. Do not taste chemicals that are in the science laboratory.

3. Always wear protective eyewear and laboratory coats while performing or observing experiments.

4. Tie back long hair to prevent it from becoming a fire hazard in the science laboratory.

5. Do not perform unauthorized experiments.

6. Do not store unnecessary personal items, such as book bags, coats, or purses, at the lab table or on the floor next to the lab table.

7. Do not remove equipment, biological specimens, or chemicals from the laboratory.

8. Do not operate lab equipment until you have been instructed about its proper use, and any safety precautions associated with that equipment.

9. Dispose of chemicals, biological materials, used supplies or equipment, and other waste materials according to the laboratory guidelines and your instructor's directions.

10. Students who are pregnant or who have any other known or suspected condition that could compromise their health or safety in the laboratory should inform their instructor. They should also check with their physician before participating in laboratory exercises.

Precautions for Working with Blood or Body Fluids

Blood and body fluids can contain viruses that cause serious and potentially deadly diseases such as acquired immunodeficiency disease (AIDS) and chronic hepatitis. For this reason, special precautions must be observed when working with blood or body fluids. This lab manual includes only one exercise that requires a blood sample, so these precautions will address blood in particular.

1. Treat any blood or body fluid that you encounter in the science laboratory as if you know that it is infectious, and take all precautions necessary to protect yourself and others from infection.

2. Work only with your own blood sample or purchased blood from a lab that has been tested and certified non-infectious.

3. When working with blood, wear protective lab garments, such as gloves, a mask, safety goggles (or a face shield), and a laboratory coat or apron.

4. Any procedure that involves blood should be performed carefully and in a hood or biological safety cabinet.

5. Laboratory disinfectant should be used on all counters and table tops before and after any procedure that involves blood. Disinfectant should also be available in case of spills during an experiment.

6. Any spills of blood should be covered with disinfectant for 20 minutes before being cleaned up.

7. Disposable waste, such as gloves, bandages, cotton balls, slides, and syringes that have been exposed to blood, should be placed in a container to be autoclaved. Broken glass or other sharp objects should be placed in a sharps container.

8. Use only single-use, disposable lancets or needles and do not use them more than once. Dispose of all single-use, disposable lancets, needles, hematocrits, or other tools that are exposed to blood in a puncture-proof sharps biohazard container in the laboratory according to institutional guidelines. A fresh solution of 10 percent bleach solution in the biohazard sharps container will provide disinfection.

9. Disinfect any reusable supplies and equipment with fresh 10 percent bleach solution and autoclave them before thoroughly washing them with soap and hot water.

10. Wash your hands immediately and thoroughly if they are contaminated with blood. Hands can be disinfected by soaking them for 20 to 30 seconds in a phenol disinfectant detergent, and then rinsing with either water or 50–70 percent alcohol for 20 to 30 seconds. Follow by scrubbing the hands with soap and rinsing for 10 to 15 seconds in running water.

Precautions for Working with Biological Materials

The following precautions apply to working with preserved biological specimens and to dissection. If fresh specimens are used, precautions for working with blood should also be observed.

1. Work with preserved specimens in a well-ventilated room. Avoid breathing the preservation fumes for prolonged periods of time. Take breaks as necessary.

2. Wear gloves and safety goggles when working with preserved specimens, including during dissections. The gloves may be latex, nitrile, or vinyl.

3. Keep a first aid kit readily available in case of skin cuts or punctures that can occur during dissection. If a cut occurs, wash the area with disinfectant soap, notify the instructor, and seek immediate medical attention in order to reduce the risk of possible infection.

4. Be careful when cleaning sharp dissection instruments to avoid injury, and dispose of damaged dissection tool properly.

Precautions for Working with Chemicals in the Science Lab

1. Be aware of safety equipment and chemical safety procedures set in place by your institution.

2. Chemicals can cause injury if they come in contact with eyes or skin, or if they are ingested. If a lab chemical is splashed into the eyes, flush with water for 15 minutes. Lab chemicals splashed on the skin can be flushed with water for five minutes. Notify your instructor and seek immediate medical attention.

3. When heating chemicals in the lab, use only glassware marked Pyrex or Kimax. Never heat a flammable liquid over or near an open flame.

4. Read chemical labels carefully before using them. Many chemical names look or sound similar.

5. Replace covers to chemical containers immediately after using them.

6. Do not point the open end of a test tube toward yourself or another person, especially if the test tube is being heated.

7. Report all accidents and spills to your instructor.

LABORATORY SCAVENGER HUNT

The purpose of this exercise is to familiarize you with the supplies and equipment that are present in the science lab. You will also be making note of the location of safety equipment and lab supplies and equipment for use in future lab exercises. This exercise can be performed individually or in groups.

Step 1: Draw a map of the science lab.

Using the graph paper provided, draw a simple map of the science laboratory. This map does not have to be precise, but it should be accurate enough to serve as a reference in the future when you want to locate a particular piece of laboratory supply or equipment. Include the location of lab counters, tables, cabinets, and shelving.

Step 2: Mark the location of safety equipment on your map.

Locate the safety equipment and first aid kit in the laboratory and mark their location on the map. Examine each piece of safety equipment in the lab and make a note to yourself about how that equipment is used in the case of an emergency. Examine the first aid kit so that you are familiar with its contents.

Step 3: Identify and locate lab equipment and supplies.

Identify the lab equipment listed below and find its storage location in the laboratory. Once you have located an item from the list, mark its storage location in the lab on your map for future reference. For items that are not stored in the science laboratory, identify the item and make a note that it will be provided by the instructor if needed. Use Figure 1-1 to identify laboratory equipment that might be unfamiliar to you.

Laboratory Scavenger Hunt List

10% bleach solution	hazardous waste container	sharps container
beaker	hot pads	spatula
beaker tongs	hotplate	stirring rod
clay triangle	medicine dropper	test tube
crucible tongs	mortar and pestle	test tube brush
dissection tools	nichrome wire	test tube holder
erlenmeyer flask	petri dishes	tripod
first aid kit	pinch clamp and utility clamp	watch glass
forceps	ring stand and ring	wire gauze
funnel	safety equipment	
graduated cylinder	safety goggles	

Common Laboratory Equipment

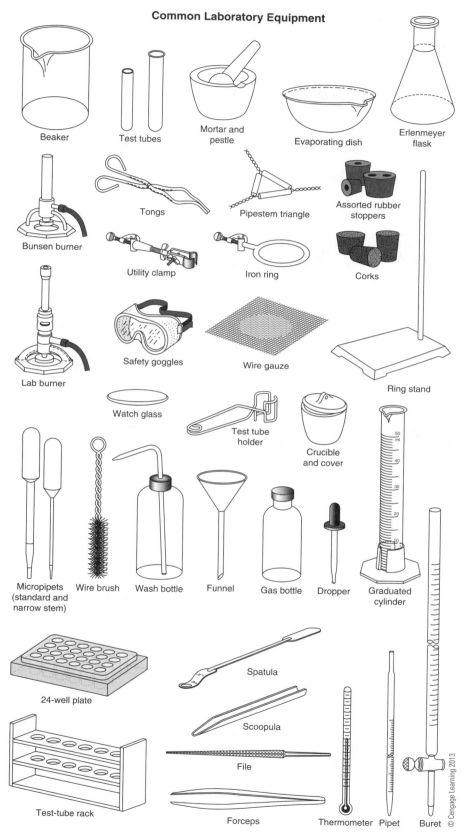

FIGURE 1-1: Laboratory Equipment

LABORATORY REPORT QUESTIONS

Long Answer

1. Where is the safety equipment in the laboratory found?

2. Where is the first aid kit in the laboratory stored?

3. What safety precautions must be taken when working with blood, blood products, or other body fluids?

4. Why is it important to assume that any blood or body fluid sample might contain infectious pathogens?

5. What precautions should be taken when working with chemicals in the laboratory?

6. What precautions should be taken when working with preserved specimens and conducting dissection?

Introduction to the Microscope and Microscopy

OBJECTIVES

At the completion of this exercise, the student should be able to:

- Demonstrate proper care of the microscope
- Identify the parts of a light microscope
- Describe the concept of magnification
- View specimens through the microscope
- Prepare a wet mount slide

MATERIALS

clean slides
cover slips
lens paper
light microscope
methylene blue dye
prepared letter "e" slides
toothpicks

INTRODUCTION

One of a scientist's most important tools is the microscope. Prior to the development of microscopes, scientists could study only structures large enough to be seen with the naked eye. Microscopes allowed for the development of whole new scientific fields—cell biology, microbiology, and histology (the study of cells and tissues of the body). While early microscopes afforded only single magnification, over time the technology has advanced dramatically. Today, microscopes range from low-magnification dissecting microscopes to exceptionally powerful electron microscopes. This lab exercise will focus on the care and use of the light microscope, the most common microscope used in college science labs.

PARTS OF A LIGHT MICROSCOPE

Though the structure of light microscopes can vary, most have the same configuration: two lenses, a platform to hold the specimen, and a light source. Figure 2-1 shows a standard light microscope and can be used to identify the parts of a light microscope.

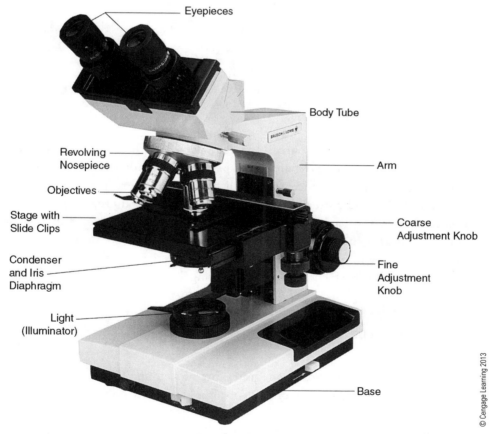

FIGURE 2-1: A standard light microscope with a mechanical stage

© Cengage Learning 2013

The **ocular** or eyepiece is a magnifying lens. Markings along the edge of the lens indicate the level of magnification, either 10X (ten times) or 15X (fifteen times). The **objective lenses** are an additional set of magnifying lenses attached to a rotating nosepiece. Each lens is labeled with its magnification. The lowest power lens—usually a 4X lens—is used for scanning slides to locate the specimen. Many microscopes will have a 10X or low dry lens instead of a scan lens. The high dry lens is usually 40X or 45X. Typically, the scan, low dry, and high dry lenses are used with only air between the slide and the objective. The highest-power lens is usually labeled "oil," "97X," or "100X" and is referred to as the oil immersion lens. This lens is used with a highly refined immersion oil that excludes air and dust. The lens should come into contact with the oil, but not touch the slide.

Microscope slides are placed on the **stage** underneath the objective lenses. The microscope in Figure 2-1 has a **mechanical stage**. A clamp holds the slide against the stage (see Figure 2-2), and two **positioning knobs** underneath the stage move the stage. Turning one positioning knob will move the slide left and right. The other moves the slide forward and back. These knobs allow a great deal of fine control when scanning the slide.

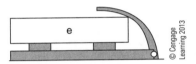

© Cengage Learning 2013

FIGURE 2-2: When using a slide clamp on a mechanical stage, the curve of the slide clamp rests against the corner of the slide to hold it in place.

In the base of the microscope is the **light source**. On some microscopes the amount of light produced by the light source can be adjusted. Between the light source and the **stage** is the **condenser,** a small circular box located below the stage. The condenser is used to concentrate the light on the **aperture**, the hole in the stage. The **iris diaphragm** is located within the condenser, and it is controlled by a small lever projecting from the condenser. Moving the lever opens or closes the diaphragm, controlling the amount of light that reaches the slide. On the sides of the microscope **body** are two knobs. The larger is the **coarse focus knob;** the smaller is the **fine focus knob.** The coarse focus knob allows large movements between the objectives and the stage. It is used initially to bring the specimen into focus. The fine focus knob is used to bring the image into sharper focus, especially with the higher power lenses.

CARE AND CLEANING OF THE MICROSCOPE

As with any other precision tool, the microscope requires careful handling. A microscope should always be carried in an upright position, holding the arm of the scope firmly in one hand and supporting the base with the other.

Use only designated lens paper to clean microscope lenses. Paper towels, tissues, and shirt sleeves can scratch the lenses, and even tiny scratches can obscure an image when magnified. Clean the oil lens last to avoid smearing immersion oil onto the other lenses. Small amounts of lens cleaner may be applied to the lens paper to remove any oil or smudges not removed by lens paper alone. Before putting the microscope away, use lens paper to clean the condenser, ocular, and objective lenses.

MAGNIFICATION AND RESOLUTION

The magnifying capability of the microscope depends on the combined power of the individual lenses. The **total magnification** of any combination of lens is calculated by multiplying the objective magnification by the ocular magnification. For example, if the ocular magnification is 5X and the objective magnification is 10X, the total will be 50X (5X multiplied by 10X).

Give a total magnification for each of the following objectives on the lab microscope:

ocular _____ × objective _____ = _____ total magnification of scanning lens

ocular _____ × objective _____ = _____ total magnification of low dry lens

ocular _____ × objective _____ = _____ total magnification of high dry lens

ocular _____ × objective _____ = _____ total magnification of oil immersion lens

A concept frequently confused with magnification is **resolution**. Resolution is the ability to distinguish two points as separate from each other. As the resolution increases, the amount of visible detail increases. At low resolution, two points that are very close together will appear as one point; at high resolution, they will be distinct from one another. Increasing the amount of available light increases resolution, whereas decreasing the light decreases resolution. **Contrast**, the difference between the lightest and darkest shades in the image, can be altered by opening or closing the iris diaphragm. Too much light decreases contrast and produces a "washed-out" image.

USING THE MICROSCOPE

When looking through the microscope, your eye should be 1 to 2 cm away from the ocular lens. The microscope may be either a monocular (one eyepiece) or binocular (two eyepieces) scope. In either case, try to keep both eyes open. This will reduce the chance of headaches and eye strain.

Gently pull the slide clamp open. Place a prepared letter "e" slide on the stage and gently close the clamp against the slide, not over it. While looking from the side, use the coarse focus knob to bring the scanning objective lens as close as possible to the slide without actually touching it. With the scanning lenses, the working distance (the space between the surface of the slide and the tip of the lens) is quite large. However, with some thick slide preparations or with the oil lens, it is possible to damage both the slide and the objective if they come in contact. The objective lenses should never touch the slide.

Next, look through the ocular and slowly turn the coarse focus knob until the specimen is clearly visible. Use the fine focus knob to fully focus the specimen. If the light is too bright or too dark, adjust the iris diaphragm. At low power, the relative size of the opening (the **field of view**) is very large, and a maximum amount of light floods the image. With higher-power objectives, the field of view narrows, less light is available, and the diaphragm needs to be adjusted to allow more light through.

While looking through the ocular, gently move the slide to the right. The image moves to the _____. Gently move the slide forward and the image moves _____. With the majority of microscopes, the images appear inverted and reversed.

To change to another objective lens, first center the image in the field of view. Remember, as the magnification increases, the field of view becomes smaller. Objects near the edge of the field will no longer be visible at higher magnification due to the smaller field of view. Once the image is centered, grasp the nose piece and turn to the next highest objective lens. Most modern microscopes are parfocal, meaning that images in focus on the lowest magnification should be in focus with minimal adjustments on the higher magnifications.

MAKING A WET MOUNT SLIDE

The letter "e" slide and the majority of slides used for histological study are permanent slides that are dried, stained, and preserved mounts that will last for years. Another, less permanent type of slide is the wet mount. As the name implies, a specimen is placed in a liquid medium, then topped with a **cover slip** before viewing. A stain is usually added to make the specimen more visible. Wet mount slides are temporary.

1. Obtain a clean cover slip and blank slide. If the slide is not clean, wash it.

2. Place a drop of dilute methylene blue stain on the slide.

3. Using a clean toothpick, gently scrape the inside of the cheek to obtain a sample of skin cells.

4. Stir the cheek cells into the drop of stain on the slide.

5. Place the cover slip perpendicular to the slide and touch the edge to the drop of stain. It should spread along the edge of the cover slip (see Figure 2-3).

6. Slowly lower the cover slip, allowing air bubbles to escape.

7. Examine the slide.

8. When finished, dispose of the slide as instructed.

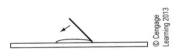

© Cengage Learning 2013

FIGURE 2-3: A cover slip should be placed on edge and lowered over the specimen at an angle to allow air bubbles to escape.

LABORATORY REPORT QUESTIONS

Multiple Choice

Circle the letter of the correct answer.

1. The correct objective to use when beginning to examine a slide with a light microscope is the _____.

    a. scan lens
    b. low dry lens
    c. high dry lens
    d. oil immersion lens

2. The amount of light passing through the slide can be controlled with the _____.

    a. mechanical stage
    b. nosepiece
    c. ocular lens
    d. iris diaphragm

3. When using the high power objective, it is best to use the _____ to adjust the focus.

    a. course focus knob

    b. fine focus knob

    c. iris diaphragm

    d. condenser

4. The ability to distinguish between two points as separate from each other is called _____.

    a. focal point

    b. focus

    c. resolution

    d. diffraction

5. Which objective offers the widest field of view?

    a. scan lens

    b. low dry lens

    c. high dry lens

    d. oil immersion lens

Matching

Match the descriptions of microscope structures in Column A with the terms in Column B.

Column A

____ 1. Platform on which the slide rests for viewing

____ 2. Used for precise focusing after initial focusing

____ 3. Used to increase the amount of light passing through the specimen

____ 4. Lens located on the superior end of the body tube

____ 5. Carries the objective lenses and rotates to change magnification

Column B

a. nosepiece

b. ocular

c. stage

d. fine focus knob

e. iris diaphragm

Long Answer

1. Explain the proper technique for transporting a microscope.

2. Define the following terms:

   field of view

   resolution

   total magnification

   contrast

3. What happens to the size of the field of view as magnification increases?

4. What would be the total magnification of a specimen if the eyepiece is 15X and the objective lens selected is 4X?

5. What is the purpose of the oil immersion lens?

6. A student is observing a specimen on the low power objective. When she switches to high power, the specimen is no longer visible. Why might this happen?

COMPARISON OF CLEANSERS— AN INTRODUCTION TO SCIENTIFIC EXPERIMENTATION

OBJECTIVES

At the completion of this exercise, the student should be able to:

- Describe the scientific method
- Identify controls and variables in an experiment
- Use sterile technique to successfully culture microbes from the skin
- Explain the role of normal flora on the skin
- Draw conclusions from experimental data

MATERIALS

four soaps or cleansers (see formulas on page 19)
incubator
permanent marker
sterile petri plate with nutrient agar
sterile swabs for sampling
sterile water
towel

INTRODUCTION

The idea behind this lab is three-fold. First, it serves as an introduction to the scientific method, the basic set of principles that governs the exploration of the world from a scientific standpoint. Second, this lab exercise introduces you to microbiology and the organisms that normally live on your skin (**normal flora**). Third, it offers a chance to conduct experiments to determine—for you—which is the best cleanser.

CULTURING BACTERIA FROM THE SKIN

The body is home to a wide range of bacteria that usually live harmlessly with us. The normal flora that live on the skin surface keep the skin clean by eating dead cells and compete with pathogenic organisms for both space and nutrients. Transient flora are microorganisms that cannot live for long on humans. They are temporary visitors acquired from the objects we come in contact with. Most humans carry a collection of such organisms on their skin. In this experiment, you are taking samples of normal skin flora and examining how different cleansers affect the number of bacteria left on the skin. The bacteria are accessed using sterile swabs and then placed in a petri dish. A solid medium in the dish, known as nutrient agar, serves as food for the bacteria.

THE SCIENTIFIC METHOD

The scientific method is a protocol for scientific investigation. It involves a series of steps that, when followed correctly, provide scientifically sound answers. The method begins with **observation**. You watch the world around you and notice something. For example, you know that if you do not wash, your skin becomes layered in dirt, feels unpleasant, and has a higher risk of infection than if it is clean. However, you also note that some cleansers make your skin feel unpleasant while others make it feel good. You also know that microbes live on your skin. You make note of what you observe and read and propose a **hypothesis**—an educated guess about your observation. In this lab experiment, you will predict which cleanser works best.

Next, you design an **experiment** to determine which cleanser is most effective. Scientific experiments have controls and variables. **Controls** are the conditions that you keep constant throughout the experiment. In this experiment, the controls will be the skin being tested, the water and towels used, and the nutrient agar in the petri dish. **Variables** are the single items that are changed, one at a time. In this experiment, the variables will be the types of cleanser used. When everyone in class compares results, another variable—the individuality of each person's skin and the normal flora that inhabit it—becomes a second, compounding variable. An experiment will typically have a detailed protocol or series of directions that attempt to control the variables. A well-designed experiment is repeatable and consistently gives the same results. If the results are not consistent, there is reason to believe something other than the variables being tested is influencing the experiment.

During the experiment, record your **data**, the results obtained from each cleanser tested. There are two major classifications of data—quantitative measures and qualitative measures. **Quantitative measures** are objective measures, such as the number of organisms on the petri plate and are typically expressed as numbers. **Qualitative measures** are more subjective. Many scientists dismiss qualitative measures as unscientific. However, they are measures of perception—an important evaluative skill for an observer. Qualitative measures include information such as your evaluation of the feel of skin of your skin after cleansing, and whether you liked the way the product smelled.

Once you have recorded the data from the experiment, it is time to **analyze the data** and **discuss the results**. How many of organisms grew on the petri dish for each treatment, and how do their numbers relate to the product's cleaning ability? Did you prefer one cleanser over the others? Your final **conclusion** determines whether your hypothesis is correct and gives further suggestions for research.

If the results are properly presented, another person should be able to repeat the experiment using the report as his or her guide.

SAMPLING

1. Gather your materials, including four skin cleaning products that you will test.

2. On the chart, record the ingredients in each product. Commercial product ingredients can be obtained from the package or the manufacturer's website.

3. Using a marker, divide the outside of the bottom of the petri plate into five equal segments (Figure 3-1).

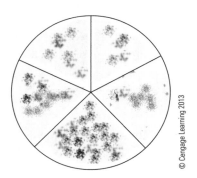

© Cengage Learning 2013

FIGURE 3-1: Using a permanent marker, divide the bottom of the outside of the dish into five sections and label each.

4. Label the sections of the dish, one for each cleanser to be tested.

5. Open the lid of the petri dish only partway to avoid contamination from the room air. Then, using a swab moistened with sterile water, streak across an area of your unwashed skin and then streak onto the plate in section 1 (Figure 3-2). The sample in section 1 is your control.

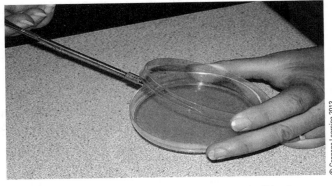

© Cengage Learning 2013

FIGURE 3-2: Avoid contaminating the petri dish; open the lid only partway when streaking a section with a cotton swab.

6. Using the cleansers of choice, follow the product's directions, using each product on a separate area of skin.

7. Moisten a new sterile swab with sterile water, then sample each cleaned area and streak it onto one of each of the four remaining sections of the petri dish.

8. Dispose of used swabs in the biohazard container.

9. Label the plate with your name and the date.

10. Invert the plate (agar side up) and incubate it for 48 hours in an incubator at 37 degrees C (98.6 degrees F).

11. After incubation, examine your petri dish and count the number and variety of colonies in each section (Figure 3-3). Record your findings in the appropriate section of the chart.

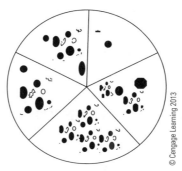

FIGURE 3-3: Colonies of bacteria appear as small masses on the surface of the agar.

© Cengage Learning 2013

RECIPES

The following are recipes for natural cleansing products that you may wish to use as skin cleansers during the experiment.

Oat, Citrus, and Almond Scrub

20 g oatmeal
20 g almonds
5 mL citrus juice
30 mL grapeseed oil
warm water

Grind the oatmeal and almonds until fine.
Add the oil and mix well.
Store in a sterile jar.
To use, combine a small amount of the mixture with warm water and use the fingertips to massage the mixture into the skin.
Rinse with warm water.

Cleansing Cream

15 mL melted beeswax
90 mL grapeseed oil
30 mL lavender or rosewater
2 drops lavender oil

Melt the wax and oil together over low heat.
Remove from heat and slowly whisk in the flower
water and lavender oil, stirring constantly.
Continue whisking until the mixture thickens and cools.
Smooth the mixture over the skin and leave it on for
15 minutes.
Rinse with warm water.

Apple and Sage Cleanser

¼ apple
15 mL glycerin
2 fresh sage leaves

Peel and cube the apple.
Grind the apple with glycerin and sage leaves with a
mortar and pestle.
Smooth the mixture over the skin and leave it on for
15 minutes.
Rinse with warm water.

Lavender Cleanser

10 g oat bran
1 g dried lavender flowers
50 mL boiling water
5 drops glycerin

Combine lavender and boiling water.
Steep 15 minutes.
Strain out the herb.
Combine the infusion with glycerin and bran to form a paste.
Cool until comfortable to the touch, then apply to skin
and scrub.
Rinse with warm water.

LAB CHART

sample	ingredients	number of colonies	comments (how does your skin look, feel, smell, etc.)
unwashed skin			
cleanser 1			
cleanser 2			
cleanser 3			
cleanser 4			

LABORATORY REPORT QUESTIONS

1. What was your original hypothesis?

2. Which cleanser was the most effective at removing microbes from the skin?

3. Why did you make that decision?

4. Did your conclusions support your hypothesis?

5. How do your results compare with those of your classmates?

Multiple Choice

Circle the letter of the correct answer.

1. The results of an experiment based on the experimental data form the _____.

    a. hypothesis
    b. quantitative measures
    c. conclusion
    d. qualitative measures

2. _____ are the bacteria that normally live on the body without causing harm.

    a. Pathogens
    b. Normal flora
    c. Hypotheses
    d. Transient flora

3. In this experiment, the bacteria you are culturing feed on _____.

    a. lavender
    b. nutrient agar
    c. soap
    d. beeswax

4. When sampling the skin, _____.

    a. one swab can be used for all the samples
    b. swabs should be shared between students
    c. a new, sterile swab is used for each sample
    d. swabs are not needed

5. Which of the following is an example of quantitative data?

   a. The cleanser made my skin flaky and red.

   b. The petri dish contained lots of red, yellow, and white colonies.

   c. The rinsed-sink section of the petri dish contains 47 colonies.

   d. The hand sanitizer smells like lilies.

Matching

Match the descriptions in Column A with the terms in Column B.

Column A	Column B
___ 1. Those factors in an experiment that are not changed	a. hypothesis
___ 2. Subjective data; information that different researchers may perceive differently	b. variable
___ 3. The test items that change over the course of an experiment	c. control
___ 4. Objective data; information that would be perceived identically by different researchers	d. qualitative data
___ 5. A statement based on observations and tested by experimentation	e. quantitative data

Long Answer

1. Why do you need to sample the unwashed skin?

2. Why is it important to sample variables one at a time?

3. Why is it a bad idea to remove all the normal flora from the skin?

4. Why do different people choose different cleansers?

ANATOMY OF THE HUMAN BODY—A SYSTEM OVERVIEW

OBJECTIVES

At the completion of this exercise, the student should be able to:

- Identify the components of the cardiovascular system
- Name the components of the respiratory system
- Identify the components of the digestive system
- Distinguish the components of the nervous system
- Identify the components of the urinary system

MATERIALS

anatomical charts
human anatomical models
  full torso
  heart
  kidney
  lungs

INTRODUCTION

The structure, or anatomy, of the body affects how it functions. One component of understanding how the body functions is knowing where the organs are located in relation to one another. Gross anatomy is the study of the structures in the body large enough to be seen with the naked eye. This lab exercise is designed to familiarize you with the gross anatomy of several of the body systems and their physical relationship to one another.

Anatomy of the Cardiovascular System

The cardiovascular system includes the heart, blood vessels, and the blood that flows through the system. The heart (Figure 4-1) consists of four chambers—two upper atria and two lower ventricles. The right and left ventricles are separated by the tricuspid valve. The bicuspid, or mitral, valve separates the left atrium and ventricle. A septum separates the left and right sides of the heart. Typically, the left ventricle has a thicker wall than the right ventricle. The cardiac muscle is supplied by the coronary vessels, which can be seen on the outside of the heart.

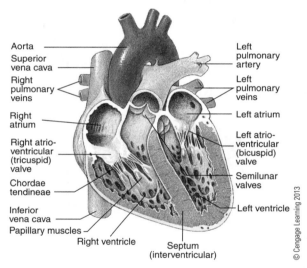

FIGURE 4-1: The structure of the heart.

© Cengage Learning 2013

Blood travels from the heart through the body in the blood vessels. In its simplest form, arteries carry blood away from the heart, and veins return it to the heart (Figure 4-2). The tiny capillaries connect arteries to veins and are the site of the exchange of materials between the blood and the tissues. Blood returning from the body has a lower level of oxygen and enters the right atrium before it flows through the tricuspid valve into the right ventricle. As the right ventricle contracts, the blood is pushed through the pulmonary arteries to the lungs, where it is oxygenated. The oxygenated blood returns to the heart through the pulmonary veins, enters the left atrium, passes through the bicuspid valve into the left ventricle, and begins its journey back out to the body through the aorta.

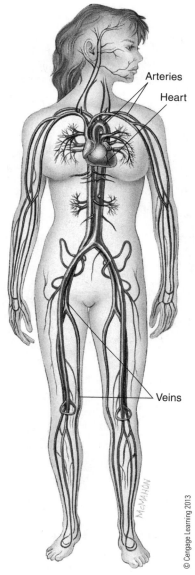

Arteries

Heart

Veins

FIGURE 4-2: The structures of the cardiovascular system.

Anatomy of the Respiratory System

The respiratory system is designed to exchange oxygen and carbon dioxide (CO_2) between the air and the blood (Figure 4-3). The nose, mouth, pharynx (back of the throat), and sinuses clean, warm, and humidify air, bringing it to body temperature and 100 percent humidity before it enters the lungs. Air travels from the upper respiratory area through the trachea to the lungs. The trachea branches into the left and right bronchi. Each bronchus branches off into increasing finer passageways until each ends at a small pocket of cells called an alveolus (plural, *alveoli).

Gas exchange occurs in the alveoli. The membrane between the capillaries and the air is thin and oxygen can diffuse easily across it into the blood. Carbon dioxide waste diffuses out of the blood and into the air in the alveoli. On exhalation, the air is forced out of the alveoli, back up the trachea, and out the nose or mouth.

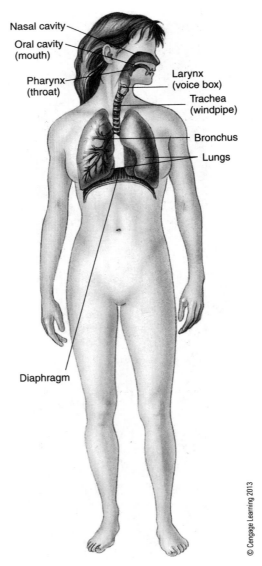

Nasal cavity

Oral cavity
(mouth)

Pharynx
(throat)

Larynx
(voice box)

Trachea
(windpipe)

Bronchus

Lungs

Diaphragm

© Cengage Learning 2013

FIGURE 4-3: The structure of the respiratory system.

Anatomy of the Digestive System

The digestive system is responsible for breaking down food, chemically breaking it into forms that can be absorbed by the body and removing the leftover waste. The majority of the digestive system consists of a hollow, muscular tube that extends from the mouth to the anus (Figure 4-4). In addition, accessory organs attached along this tube contribute to digestion and nutrient processing.

The teeth grind food into smaller pieces, making it easier to swallow. As food is chewed, it is moistened by saliva, which contains enzymes, bicarbonate buffer, and water. The addition of saliva makes food easier to swallow and begins breaking down starches into simple sugars. Chewing increases the surface area of the food, making it easier for enzymes to break down the food chemically.

The esophagus is a tube that connects the mouth to the stomach. When swallowing, the smooth muscle of the esophagus uses peristaltic waves to push the food along. Between the esophagus and the stomach, food must pass the esophageal sphincter, a ring of smooth muscle that controls movement into the stomach.

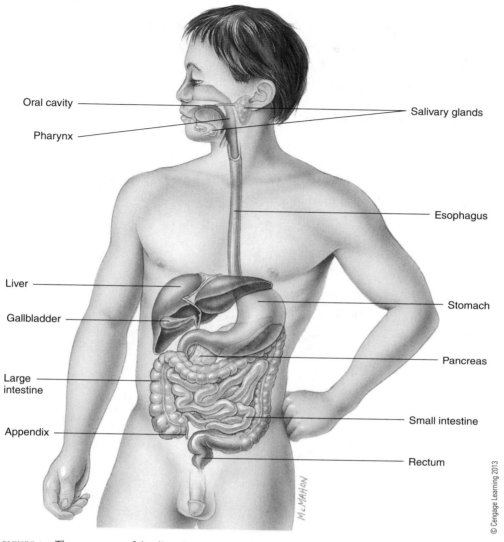

Oral cavity

Pharynx

Salivary glands

Esophagus

Liver

Gallbladder

Stomach

Pancreas

Large intestine

Small intestine

Appendix

Rectum

McMAHON

© Cengage Learning 2013

FIGURE 4-4: The structures of the digestive system.

The stomach is a muscular pouch lined with a mucous membrane. The chewed food is combined with stomach secretions to become chyme. Stomach secretions include hydrochloric acid which kills microbes and denature proteins, the enzyme pepsin that digests proteins, several hormones, and the name of the chemical is intrinsic factor that helps the intestines absorb vitamin B_{12}. The stomach acts as a holding area. When the stomach stretches with chyme, it sends the brain a "full" signal that alerts it to stop eating. From the stomach, measured amounts of chyme pass through the pyloric sphincter and enter the small intestine. In the first few inches of the small intestine, pancreatic juice (consisting of a substance called bicarbonate and the enzymes trypsin, lipase, and amylase) adjusts the pH of the chyme to neutral. Two pancreatic enzymes—trypsin and amylase—are added to the chyme to digest protein and starch, respectively. Bile from the gall bladder is also added and acts as a detergent, breaking apart fats so that they can be digested by the enzyme lipase. Further along in the small intestines, nutrients from the digested food are absorbed. Water-soluble nutrients, such as sugars and amino acids, move into the bloodstream. Fat-soluble nutrients and lipids move into the lymphatic system and are returned to the blood near the heart. The large intestine absorbs water, holds waste, and is home to a collection of normal flora. The waste materials move through the large intestine and are held there until defecation.

While not directly connected to the digestive system, the liver is an integral part of the system. Bile is made in the liver cells (hepatocytes) and stored in the gall bladder, which is located on the underside of the liver. The hepatocytes remove waste materials and convert many toxins into less toxic forms. The blood supply from the small intestines drains into the liver before returning to the rest of the body. Microbes can be removed, toxins filtered out, and nutrient processing occurs. Fats and carbohydrates (glycogen) can be stored in the liver to provide an energy reserve. The liver is involved in breaking down protein, fats and carbohydrates. Plasma proteins involved in blood clotting are produced there as well.

Anatomy of the Nervous System

The nervous system consists of the brain, spinal cord, and peripheral nerves (Figure 4-5). The sensory nerves respond to a stimulus and transmit a nerve impulse to the spinal cord. The spinal cord carries the impulse to the brain, where information is processed. Both the brain and spinal cord are encased in bone. Signals from the brain travel down the spinal cord and through the motor nerves to muscle and glands.

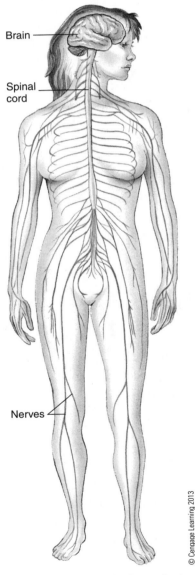

© Cengage Learning 2013

FIGURE 4-5: The nervous system—brain, spinal cord, and nerves.

Anatomy of the Urinary System

The urinary system includes a pair of kidneys that are located against the back wall of the abdominal cavity (Figure 4-6). Each kidney filters blood, removes wastes, and balances electrolytes to produce urine. As urine is produced, it passes through muscular tubes called ureters, to the bladder for storage. The bladder is located low in the pelvic cavity. In females, the uterus curves over the top of the bladder. From the bladder, urine exits the body through the urethra.

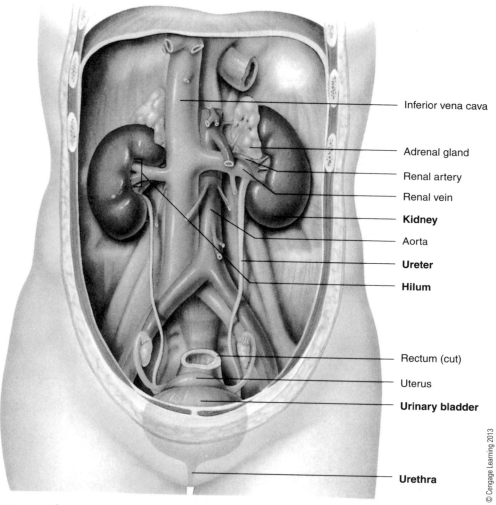

FIGURE 4-6: The structure of the urinary system.

© Cengage Learning 2013

PROCEDURES

1. Identify each of the following structures on the charts and models:

   arteries

   bladder

   brain

bronchi

esophagus

gall bladder

heart

    left atrium

    left ventricle

    right atrium

    right ventricle

kidney

large intestine

liver

lungs

nerves

pancreas

small intestine

spinal cord

stomach

trachea

ureter

urethra

veins

LABORATORY REPORT QUESTIONS

Multiple Choice

Circle the letter of the correct answer.

1. In the respiratory, gas exchange occurs in the _____.
    a. alveoli
    b. bronchi
    c. trachea
    d. sinuses

2. The liver is located below the _____.

   a. small intestine
   b. gall bladder
   c. lungs
   d. trachea

3. The _____ connects the stomach to the large intestine.

   a. liver
   b. pancreas
   c. small intestine
   d. trachea

4. Bile is produced in the _____.

   a. stomach
   b. pancreas
   c. liver
   d. gall bladder

5. Partially digested food leaving the stomach enters the _____.

   a. arteries
   b. liver
   c. small intestine
   d. alveoli

Matching

Match the descriptions in Column A with the structures in Column B.

Column A	Column B
___ 1. Adds digestive enzymes to the small intestine	a. ureter
___ 2. Carries impulses to the brain and sensory nerves	b. left atrium
___ 3. Heart chamber that receives blood from the lungs	c. pancreas
___ 4. Connects the kidney to the bladder	d. esophagus
___ 5. Connects the mouth to the stomach	e. spinal cord

Long Answer

1. How do the respiratory and cardiovascular systems work together?

2. Describe the path a nerve impulse travels, from when a finger touches a warm surface to the muscle contracting and the hand is withdrawn.

3. What structures does blood pass through, between entering the heart through the right atrium and exiting the heart through the aorta?

4. Where is the gall bladder located in relation to the liver?

5. How does the urinary system coordinate with the cardiovascular system?

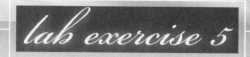

SKELETAL SYSTEM—DIFFERENCES BETWEEN WOMEN AND MEN

OBJECTIVES

At the completion of this exercise, the student should be able to:

- Identify whether a skeleton is male or female
- Identify the location of the bones on yourself
- Describe the structural differences between male and female skeletons
- Identify several of the bones that make up the skeleton
- Identify the structures that comprise the microanatomy of the bone tissues
- Describe the roles that osteoblasts, osteoclasts, and osteocytes play in maintaining bone density

MATERIALS

lens paper
microscope
prepare microscope slide of ground bone
skeleton model

INTRODUCTION

The skeleton provides a framework to support and protect the other organs. The skeleton consists of the bones plus the ligaments and cartilage that holds the bones together. The skeleton is designed to protect fragile and essential organs and to provide support for the body. Muscles attach to the bones and act as pulleys for movement. In addition, the bones act as storage sites for minerals and fat, and house the bone marrow, which produces blood cells.

Although similar, male and female skeletons do show some predictable differences that can be used to distinguish them. In addition, the physiology of the bone tissues themselves contribute to the differences in bone densities found in men and women and to their susceptibility to osteoporosis later in life.

GROSS ANATOMY OF THE SKELETON

Before examining differences between male and female skeletons, it is useful to know the names and locations of the major bones. The skeleton can be divided into two major areas: the axial skeleton and the appendicular skeleton. The axial skeleton consists of the skull, vertebrae, sternum, and ribs. It shelters the essential organs such as the brain, heart, and lungs, protecting them from potential injury. The appendicular skeleton is primarily involved in movement. The major bones of both components are identified in Figure 5-1.

Locate the following bones in Figure 5-1. Next, identify the bones on the skeleton models.

skull

clavicle

scapula

sternum

pelvis

vertebrae

rib

carpals

femur

humerus

tarsals

Notice how bones are attached to each other, and the degree of flexibility the attachments allow. The attachments between bones are called **articulations**. Most articulations include ligaments, which are strong, flexible bands of collagen that attach one bone to the bone next to it, while some articulations include less flexible fibrous connections between bones. In general, these articulations represent a compromise between strength and flexibility. For example, the articulations between the bones that comprise the skull are strong and relatively rigid to protect the brain. Other joints, such as the knee or ankle joints, provide much more movement but are also more vulnerable to damage resulting in strains and sprains.

During the last weeks of pregnancy, a hormone called relaxin allows the ligaments in the skeleton to stretch more than usual, which will allow more flexibility in the pelvic joints as the infant moves through the birth canal during parturition. This increased flexibility, however, affects all of the joints and can contribute to the characteristic "waddle" of late-term pregnancy.

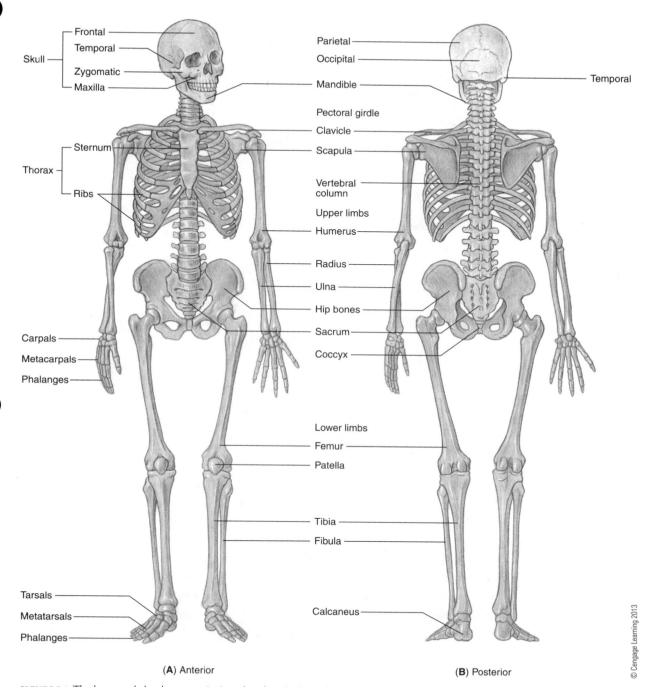

Skull
— Frontal
— Temporal
— Zygomatic
— Maxilla

Thorax
— Sternum
— Ribs

Carpals
Metacarpals
Phalanges

Tarsals
Metatarsals
Phalanges

Parietal
Occipital
Mandible
Temporal
Pectoral girdle
Clavicle
Scapula
Vertebral column
Upper limbs
Humerus
Radius
Ulna
Hip bones
Sacrum
Coccyx

Lower limbs
Femur
Patella

Tibia
Fibula

Calcaneus

(A) Anterior   **(B)** Posterior

© Cengage Learning 2013

FIGURE 5-1: The human skeletal system. A. Anterior view. B. Posterior view.

SKELETAL DIFFERENCES BETWEEN FEMALES AND MALES

There are several differences between the male and female skeleton, chiefly in the pelvis, femur, knee joint, and elbow (Figure 5-2). These differences are related to childbearing. The pelvis of a woman is wider than that of a man, and is tipped slightly, allowing the maximum opening at the pelvic outlet. Examine the male pelvis. Now try and imagine a baby's head fitting through the pelvic opening. In addition, the **subpubic angle**—the angle under the pubic symphysis—is greater than 90 degrees in a woman and less than 90 degrees in a male.

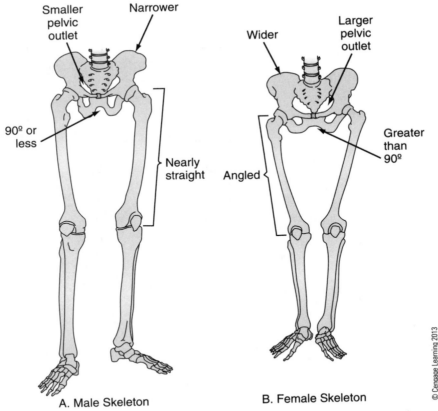

FIGURE 5-2: A & B. The primary differences between the male and female skeleton can be seen in the pelvic bones and femur.

The difference in the width of the pelvis alters the angle of a woman's femur and knee joint, making it different from that of a male. A man's femur is oriented nearly vertically from the hip to the knee and articulates perpendicularly to the tibia. If this orientation occurred in a woman, the width of the pelvis would make it impossible for her to bring her feet together. To compensate for the wider pelvis, a woman's femur angles inward and articulates at an angle with the tibia. This angle is called the quadraceps (Q) angle. The increased Q angle in women can create additional stress on the knees, and shifts a woman's posture compared to that of a man.

In addition, a woman's humerus is held at a different angle than a man's, also due to the wider width of a woman's hips. Unless a woman also has wide shoulders, her arms cannot hang straight down without hitting her hips. To compensate, most women hold their elbows at a slight angle. In addition, males have proportionately longer forearms than females do.

MICROANATOMY OF THE SKELETON

Bone tissue consists of living cells and a non-living solid matrix made up of collagen protein and calcium-rich minerals. When viewed under the microscope, the matrix resembles a series of concentric circles similar to the growth rings in a tree stump. These concentric rings are called the **lamella**, and they comprise the Haversian system. At the center of each group of lamella is a Haversian canal, which contains the blood vessels and nerves. Each group of lamella and Haversian canal is referred to as an **osteon**. Within each osteon, the lamella is bordered by lacuna, or spaces filled with bone cells.

Three types of bone cells are active in the bone tissue. **Osteoclasts** move through the bone tissue, destroying older bone matrix so that it can be regularly replaced with fresh bone tissue. **Osteoblasts** follow the osteoclasts, depositing new collagen and mineral to form new matrix. On average, the activities of osteoclasts and osteoblasts are balanced and the density of the bones remains constant. **Osteocytes** are mature bone osteoblasts that reside in the lacuna and maintain the bone tissues.

The activities of the osteoclasts, osteoblasts, and osteocytes are regulated by several hormones, including some sex hormones like estrogen and testosterone. These hormones stimulate the activities of osteoblasts and are important for maintaining bone density. As men and women age and their sex hormone levels decline, the activities of the osteoclasts outpace those of the osteoblasts. This effect is more pronounced in women and can result in a decline in bone density and the higher incidence of osteoporosis in women than in men.

Identify the following components of the bone tissue in the Figure 5-3 and in a prepared ground bone microscope slide.

lamella

lacunae

osteon

Haversian canal

mineralized matrix

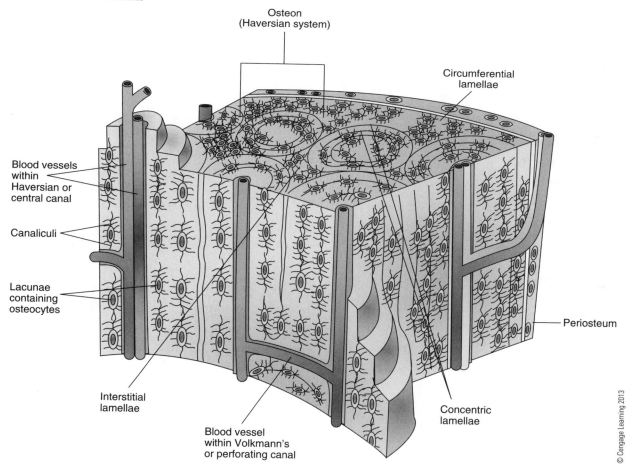

FIGURE 5-3: The microscopic structure of bone.

© Cengage Learning 2013

LABORATORY REPORT QUESTIONS

Multiple Choice

Circle the letter of the correct answer.

1. The largest bone in the leg is the _____.

   a. tibula
   b. femur
   c. humerus
   d. tarsus

2. Which type of bone is found in both the arm and the leg?

   a. humerus
   b. vertebrae
   c. sacrum
   d. phalanges

3. Which of these is often referred to as the "collar bone"?

   a. sternum
   b. scapula
   c. clavicle
   d. sacrum

4. Which angle is usually greater in females than in males?

   a. sub-pubic angle
   b. sub-sacral angle
   c. Q angle
   d. angle of the clavicle

5. Which of these creates new bone tissue?

   a. osteoclasts
   b. osteoblasts
   c. osteocytes
   d. lacuna

Matching

Match the descriptions in Column A with the structures in Column B.

Column A	Column B
B 1. Series of concentric lamella and the Haversian canal	a. lacuna
E 2. Mature bone cell	b. osteon
D 3. Non-living mineralized material	c. lamella
A 4. Space where osteocytes reside	d. matrix
C 5. Layers of matrix	e. osteocyte

Long Answer

1. Explain how articulations represent a compromise between strength and flexibility.

2. Define the following terms:

   Q angle

   pubic symphysis

   tendon

   matrix

3. How do osteoclasts and osteoblasts maintain bone density and contribute to bone health?

4. How can male and female skeletons be distinguished from each other?

The ~~From~~ Females

5. How might differences in skeletal characteristics between men and women affect their posture, or how they move?

BLOOD

At the completion of this exercise, the student should be able to:

- Identify the components of blood
- Describe the role of erythrocytes
- Describe the role of platelets
- Describe the role of the white blood cells
- Explain what a differential WBC count measures
- Explain what a hematocrit measures

centrifuge
clay for hematocrit
hematocrit
lancet
lens paper
light microscope
prepared human blood microscope slides

INTRODUCTION

Blood provides oxygen and nutrients to our cells and removes waste materials. The white blood cells battle pathogens to keep us healthy. It helps us maintain homeostasis, keeping the body in balance. Blood accounts for seven to eight percent of the body's weight, and the average person has approximately four to five liters of blood. The normal pH of blood ranges between 7.35 and 7.45, just slightly alkaline, maintained at this pH by a number of buffers in the blood. Blood has many different components, and the relative percentages of these components are an indicator of health status.

THE COMPONENTS OF BLOOD

Blood is composed of plasma and formed elements (Figure 6-1). Plasma consists of 90 percent water; the rest of the volume is dissolved proteins, electrolytes, minerals, and other substances. Plasma proteins include the antibodies that fight infections, fibrinogen (a clotting factor), enzymes, hormones, and albumin. The formed elements are suspended in the plasma and include platelets, red blood cells (erythrocytes), and white blood cells (leukocytes).

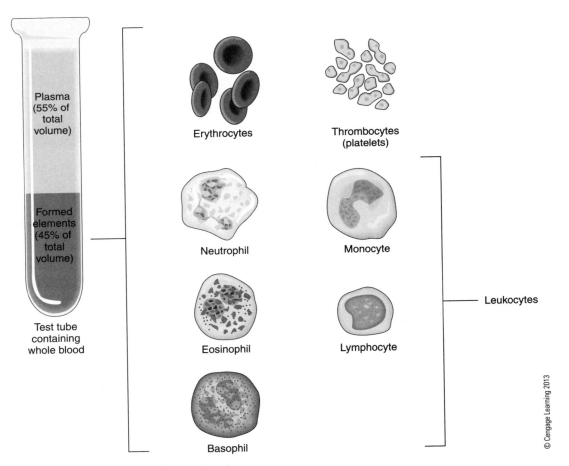

© Cengage Learning 2013

FIGURE 6-1: The composition of human blood.

The Formed Elements

Red blood cells (RBC) carry oxygen throughout the body. A mature red blood cell has no nucleus. Its color is due to an iron-rich molecule called hemoglobin. Women typically have four to five million RBCs per cubic millimeter of blood. For men, the concentration is higher, 4.5 million to 6 million per cubic millimeter. Men and women also vary in the level of hemoglobin in their blood. Women average 12 to 16 g/dl of hemoglobin while men average 14 to 18 g/dl. Their lower average hemoglobin levels make women more prone to a medical condition called anemia.

Platelets are fragments of immature blood cells called megakaryocytes. Platelets travel through the bloodstream. When they come into contact with collagen fibers—most often due to damaged blood vessels—platelets stick together to begin the process of forming a blood clot. Platelet numbers vary from 150,000 to 400,000 per cubic millimeter of blood.

White blood cells (WBC) primarily serve an immune function, and their relative numbers in the blood indicate immune health and the presence or absence of infection. There are several kinds of white blood cells. Neutrophils comprise 50 to 70 percent of white blood cells. Their role is phagocytic—that is, they engulf invading bacteria, viruses, and other abnormal cells. Neutrophils are most easily identified by their highly irregular nucleus and the pale granules in their cytoplasm.

Macrophages, another type of phagocytic cell, are larger than neutrophils, often have a bean-shaped nucleus, and have no granules in their cytoplasm. Macrophages may remain in the bloodstream or migrate into the tissues. Some organs contain fixed macrophages—macrophages that always remain on patrol there. Such macrophages include Kupffer cells in the liver, microglia in the nervous system, and alveolar macrophages in the lungs.

Eosinophils have a granular cytoplasm. Their name is derived from the ability of their granules to absorb eosin dye, which gives them a pinkish-orange color when viewed under the microscope. Although eosinophils typically account for only about two to four percent of white blood cells, during chronic allergic reactions or parasitic worm infections, they may skyrocket to more than 50 percent of the white blood cell count.

Another type of leukocyte is basophils. Because granules in basophil cytoplasm absorb a blue dye, they appear blue under the microscope, with heavily dyed granules sometimes so plentiful that they obscure the nucleus. Basophils account for less than one percent of the white blood cells in the human body. They secrete histamine and other chemicals involved in the inflammation response.

Lymphocytes are a specialized type of white blood cell, making up 20 to 30 percent of the leukocytes in the blood. Their numbers can increase dramatically during infections. Lymphocytes are the source of antibodies, specialized proteins that destroy bacteria and viruses that could cause disease. Because lymphocytes also store an immunological memory of previous infections, the body can respond quickly if it encounters a particular kind of disease organism more than once. This immune memory minimizes the possibility of reinfection with the same pathogen.

DIFFERENTIAL WBC COUNT

A differential white blood cell count is a tool used to determine the ratio of the different types of white blood cells. Different types of medical conditions can alter these ratios in predictable patterns, and a differential count is a useful tool for diagnosis. During this lab exercise, the differential WBC count will be used to identify the types of white blood cells present in an average sample of blood. In this case, the average blood sample will be represented by a prepared human blood slide, viewed under the microscope.

Conducting the Differential WBC Count

For this exercise, work in groups of four students. Each group should obtain four human blood slides and label them 1-4. To conduct the differential WBC count for each slide, 100 white blood cells on a slide are examined and classified according to WBC type. Use the photographs and descriptions provided in this laboratory exercise to identify the WBCs. Each group member should conduct a differential WBC count for each of the four microscope slides and record the results in Table 6-1.

Shortcut: Instead of counting 100 WBCs, students can tally the first 50 WBCs they encounter, then multiply each count by two to find the average percentages of the individual WBC types in their samples.

TABLE 6-1: Differential WBC Count Data

WBC Type	Slide 1	Slide 2	Slide 3	Slide 4
Neutrophil				
Lymphocyte				
Eosinophil				
Basophil				
Macrophage				

TABLE 6-2: Average Values for Differential WBC Counts

WBC Type	Average Percentage
Neutrophil	60%–70%
Lymphocyte	20%–25%
Eosinophil	2%–4%
Basophil	0.5%–1%
Macrophage	3%–8%

© Cengage Learning 2013

How average were the sample counts? Group members can compare their individual data to determine the level of variability in the results. They can also compare their results to standardized results displayed in Table 6-2. Were any of the differential WBC counts out of the ordinary? If so, what information does the abnormal count give about potential conditions that may be present?

HEMATOCRIT

A hematocrit is a method used to determine approximate RBC volumes. To test hematocrit, a finger is pricked with a sterile lance and a few drops of blood drawn into a capillary tube. The end of the tube is sealed with wax or clay, and the sample centrifuged. Centrifuging causes the blood components to separate into layers, and the RBCs, being heaviest, settle to the bottom of the tube. The WBCs form the next layer, called a buffy coat due to its color. The top of the tube contains the plasma. A hematocrit is determined by dividing the height of RBCs by the height of the total blood column, including the plasma on top. Average values for men range from 42 to 52. For women, who have fewer RBCs, the value is usually between 37 and 47. Hematocrits that fall below average suggest anemia. Hematocrit values above normal may indicate polycythemia, a condition in which the body produces too many RBCs, or dehydration.

Important note: If hematocrit measurements are taken in the laboratory, the List of Precautions for Working with Blood and Body fluids from Lab Exercise 1 Lab Safety must be reviewed and adhered to.

LABORATORY REPORT QUESTIONS

Multiple Choice

Circle the letter of the correct answer.

1. Which of these are found in plasma?

   a. water
   b. dissolved protein
   c. electrolytes
   d. all of the above

2. What is the role of red blood cells?

   a. They initiate clot formation to stop bleeding.
   b. They contain hemoglobin to transport oxygen.
   c. These fight infection.
   d. All of the above

3. Which of these secretes histamine, a substance that causes inflammation?

   a. eosinophils
   b. erythrocytes
   c. basophils
   d. macrophages

4. Which WBC type produces antibodies?

   a. lymphocytes
   b. neutrophils
   c. basophils
   d. macrophages

5. A low hematocrit number could indicate _____.

   a. an infection
   b. dehydration
   c. anemia
   d. blood loss due to injury

Matching

Match the descriptions in Column A with the structures in Column B.

Column A

___ 1. Red blood cells

___ 2. White blood cell that combats parasitic worm infections

___ 3. White blood cell that can migrate out of the bloodstream into the tissues

___ 4. General phagocyte

___ 5. General term for a white blood cell

Column B

a. eosinophils

b. macrophage

c. neutrophils

d. erythrocyte

e. leukocyte

Long Answer

1. Describe the components of a hematocrit. What can a hematocrit indicate about health?

2. Define the following terms:

anemia

phagocytic cell

polycythemia

hemoglobin

3. Describe the components of the blood.

4. What are the roles of each type of white blood cell?

5. How do platelets help to maintain homeostasis?

6. Why are there many different kinds of white blood cells?

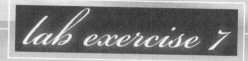

FEMALE REPRODUCTIVE SYSTEM

OBJECTIVES

At the completion of this exercise, the student should be able to:

- Identify the name and location of the major organs of the female reproductive system
- Describe the functions of the major organs of the female reproductive system
- Identify the positions and functions of the major ligaments that maintain the position of the female reproductive organs
- Describe the layers of the uterus and their functions

MATERIALS

anatomical models of female reproductive organs
dissection tray and dissection tools (if preserved specimens are available)
gloves (if preserved specimens are available)
lens paper
light microscope
prepared microscope slides of ovary
preserved specimens of human or animal reproductive organs (optional)

INTRODUCTION

The purpose of this lab exercise is to become familiar with the organs that comprise the female reproductive tract. The female reproductive system consists of the following internal structures: a pair of ovaries, their associated fallopian tubes, the uterus, and the vagina. Unlike the male reproductive tract, which joins the urethra before exiting the body, the female system has its own external genitalia, or vulva. The female system functions to produce eggs (oogenesis), to produce hormones, and to nurture the developing embryo.

VULVA AND VAGINA

In women, the external genitals consist of the vulva, which is subdivided into the labia majora, labia minora, vestibule, and clitoris. The labia majora are the outer lips of the vulva, and the labia minora are the smaller, inner lips. Pubic hair is present on the labia majora of adult females, though not on the labia minora. The vestibule is the space enclosed by the labia majora, and both the vagina and the urethra open into it.

Much of the clitoris is internal and plays an important role in sexual function. The external portion of the clitoris is located at the anterior edge of the vestibule, and it is usually covered by an extension of tissue called the clitoral hood. The clitoris contains erectile tissues and responds to stimulation by enlarging and becoming erect.

UTERUS AND CERVIX

The uterus is a pear-shaped, hollow organ. The upper portion of the uterus, where the fallopian tubes attach, is called the fundus. The fundus narrows slightly to form the body of the uterus. The cervix is the narrowest and most inferior point, and joins the uterus to the vagina. The outer surface of the uterus is continuous with the peritoneum and the ligaments which support the ovary, and is called the perimetrium. In addition, the round ligament attaches the uterus to the anterior abdominal wall. The perimetrium overlies the muscular layers of the uterus, the myometrium. The innermost layer of the uterus, the endometrium, is composed of epithelial tissues that are rich in both glands and blood supply. It is into the endometrium that a fertilized embryo implants to establish a pregnancy.

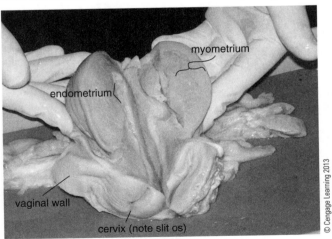

FIGURE 7-1: The interior of the human uterus.

Although the cervix is a continuation of the uterus, it is often described as a distinct structure. The cervical canal provides a passageway between the vagina and the uterus, and it is surrounded externally by a strong, thick ring of smooth muscle. The external cervical os is the opening of the cervical canal into the vagina and the internal cervical os is the opening of the canal into the uterus.

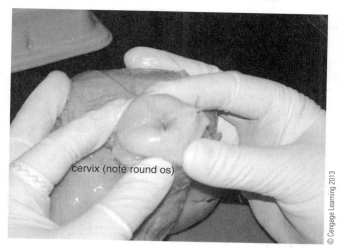

FIGURE 7-2: The human cervix.

If you compare the cervix shown in Figure 7-2 with the one in Figure 7-1, you will notice the shape of the os is different. The round os indicates this woman had never had a pregnancy (nulliparous). The os of the cervix in Figure 7-1 is elongated. This indicates that, at some point, the cervix was dilated—for example, to accommodate the delivery of a baby. After dilation, the cervical os does not return to its original round shape.

OVARIES

The ovaries produce eggs and secrete the hormones estrogen and progesterone. The ovaries usually lie against the posterior, lateral wall of the pelvic cavity. Each ovary is supported by several ligaments. The suspensory ligament contains the circulatory and nerve supply for the ovary. An ovarian ligament attaches each ovary to the lateral margin of the uterus. The broad ligament forms a flat sheet that supports both the uterus and the ovaries. A fibrous layer called the tunica albuginea covers each ovary. In a cross-section, numerous ovarian follicles are imbedded in the connective tissue (the stroma), which forms the interior of the ovaries. The germinal epithelium is located directly beneath the tunica albuginea, where the egg-containing follicles develop and secrete estrogen.

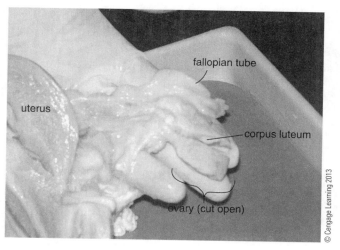

FIGURE 7-3: The position of the ovary in relation to the fallopian tube. The ovary has been cut to show a corpus luteum.

FALLOPIAN TUBES

The fallopian tubes provide a passageway for eggs to travel to the uterus, and for sperm to travel toward an egg. The end of the fallopian tube closest to the ovary is called the infundibulum. Eggs leave the ovary during ovulation and are funneled into the fallopian tubes by the fimbria which expand and surround the opening. The ovary is not in direct physical contact with the fimbria; rather, the fimbria cage the ovary. The rhythmic waving of the fimbria move the oocyte into the fallopian tube. Past the infundibulum, the tubes narrow to form the isthmus. A combination of peristaltic contraction of the smooth muscle in the walls of the fallopian tubes and currents generated by the cilia on the cells lining the tubes are believed to propel the egg toward the uterus. If fertilization occurs, it will usually take place in the distal ends of the fallopian tubes.

IDENTIFY STRUCTURES OF THE FEMALE REPRODUCTIVE SYSTEM

Identify the location and function of the following structures on Figures 7-4 and 7-5.

external genitals

- vulva
- labia majora and labia minora
- clitoris
- vestibule

vagina

uterus

- perimetrium
- endometrium
- myometrium
- cervix
- cervical os
- fundus
- fallopian tube
- ampulla
- infundibulum

fimbria

ovary

   After identifying the structures on Figures 7-4 and 7-5, identify the same structures on an anatomical model or preserved specimen.

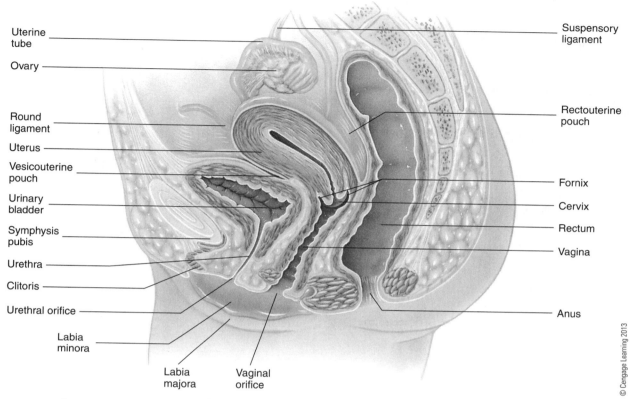

FIGURE 7-4: The organs of the female reproductive system.

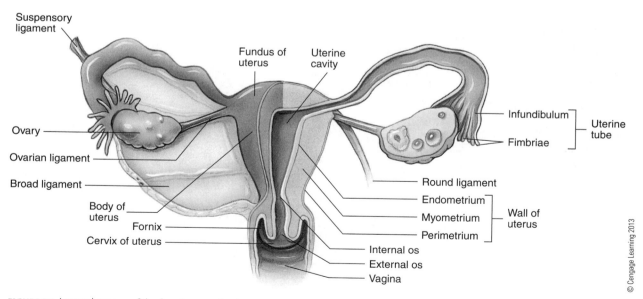

FIGURE 7-5: Internal organs of the female reproductive system.

LABORATORY REPORT QUESTIONS

Multiple Choice

Circle the letter of the correct answer.

1. What is the function of the tunica albuginea?

    a. forms the lining of the vagina
    b. prevents sperm from entering the fallopian tubes
    c. forms the outer cell layer of the ovary
    d. protects the clitoris

2. Which organ of the female reproductive system is responsible for the secretion of estrogen?

    a. vagina
    b. uterus
    c. fallopian tube
    d. ovary

3. If fertilization occurs, it will take place in the _____.

    a. vagina
    b. uterus
    c. fallopian tube
    d. ovary

4. Which of these is part of the uterus?

    a. fundus
    b. isthmus
    c. infundibulum
    d. follicle

5. Which is the muscular layer of the uterus?

    a. endometrium
    b. myometrium
    c. perimetrium
    d. cervix

Matching

Match the descriptions in Column A with the structures in Column B.

Column A	Column B
_d_ 1. Eggs travel through this structure to the uterus	a. clitoris
_b_ 2. Implantation occurs here	b. endometrium
_c_ 3. Opening of the fallopian tube	c. ampulla
_e_ 4. Follicles develop here	d. fallopian tube
_a_ 5. Contains erectile tissues	e. ovary

Long Answer

1. Describe the functions of the three layers of the uterus.

2. Define the following terms:

   cervical os

   infundibulum

   fimbria

   vestibule

3. Describe the major ligaments that support the reproductive organs.

4. Trace the path that sperm would travel as they move through the female reproductive tract. Which structures and organs would they encounter?

5. How is an egg transported to the uterus?

FEMALE REPRODUCTIVE ANATOMY UNDER THE MICROSCOPE

OBJECTIVES

At the completion of this exercise, the student should be able to:

- Identify the microanatomy of the ovary
- Describe the stages of follicular development
- Identify the microanatomy of the uterus

MATERIALS

microscope
prepared slides of the following:
   fallopian tube
   ovary
   uterus

INTRODUCTION

In its simplest terms, the ovary consists of egg follicles embedded in connective tissue. The entire structure is wrapped in a layer of fibrous connective tissue, the *tunica albuginea* (Figure 8-1).

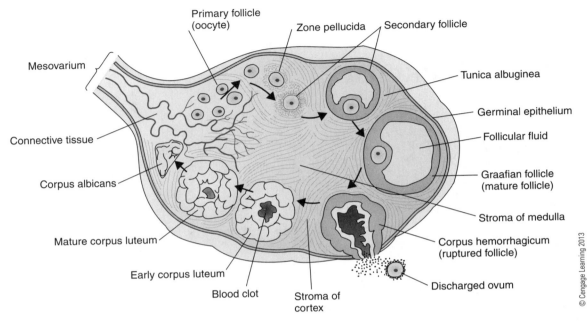

FIGURE 8-1: Microanatomy of the ovary.

Directly beneath the tunica albuginea, the germinal epithelium is visible (Figure 8-2). As the primordial follicles, or oocytes, begin to mature, they enlarge to become primary follicles. At this point, a single layer of epithelial tissue can be seen surrounding the oocyte. These cells produce estrogen.

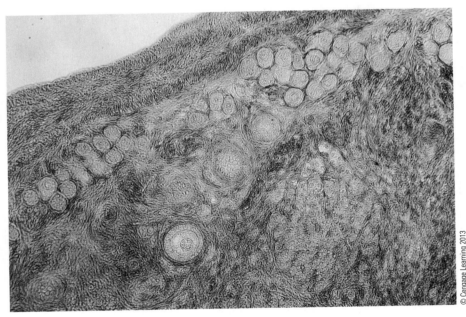

FIGURE 8-2: Germinal epithelium.

The next stage of development is the secondary follicular stage. Here, the epithelial layers surrounding the oocyte have increased in size. A fluid-filled antrum develops around the oocyte. Within this follicle a viscous layer of sugary protein and loose epithelial cells (the *zona pellucida*) can be seen surrounding the oocyte within the antrum (Figure 8-3).

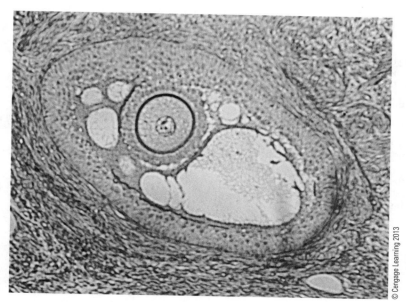

FIGURE 8-3: Secondary follicle.

Just before it is released from the ovary, the mature oocyte and its surrounding epithelial tissues are called a *graafian follicle*. Under the influence of two hormones, follicle-stimulating hormone (FSH) and luteinizing hormone (LH), the antrum continues to enlarge and additional layers within the follicle become visible. A fibrous layer, the *theca externa*, surrounds the outside of the follicle and is in contact with the stroma. The interior wall of the follicle is the *theca interna,* which secretes steroids. Deep within the theca interna are the granulosa cells, which convert the steroids from the theca interna into estrogen and are responsible for the secretion of the follicular fluid within the antrum.

When a graafian follicle ruptures at ovulation, the oocyte and its zona pellucida burst from the ovarian surface. The remnants of the follicle—the granulosa and theca cells—form a structure called the corpus luteum, which produces both estrogen and progesterone. If the oocyte is not fertilized and hormonal signals are not sent, the corpus luteum degenerates into a nonfunctional scar, the corpus albicans. If fertilization does occur, the corpus luteum will continue to produce hormones to support the establishment of the pregnancy.

As the egg is released from the ovary, it enters the fallopian tube. The outer layer of the fallopian tube is the *serosa,* a layer of flattened epithelial tissue. Beneath the serosa is the muscularis layer which is composed of smooth muscle. Contractions of the fallopian tube are thought to help move the egg through the tube toward the uterus. The inner layer of the fallopian tubes is mucosa. The mucosa is highly folded and lined with both ciliated epithelium and secretory cells. The movement of the cilia moves the egg through the tube. The secretory cells are involved in the capacitation of sperm as they move through the fallopian tubes toward the egg.

From the fallopian tube, the egg enters the uterus. The outer surface of the uterus is the perimetrium and is continuous with the peritoneum and the ligaments that support the uterus and ovaries. Beneath this layer is the myometrium, three intertwined layers of smooth muscle responsible for uterine contractions. The innermost layer of the uterus, the endometrium, is composed of epithelial tissue rich in both glands and blood supply. The endometrium itself is divided into two layers. The stratum basale is the deepest layer of epithelial tissue and is attached to the myometrium. As the stratum basale divides, the cells are pushed toward the uterine lumen and form the stratum functionalis. It is into the stratum functionalis of the endometrium that an embryo implants during pregnancy, and it is the stratum functionalis that is shed during menstruation.

PROCEDURES

Histology of the Ovary

1. Using Figures 8-1, 8-2, and 8-3 as guides, locate the following structures on the slides of the ovary. Note: Not all follicular stages may be visible on a single slide.

   antrum

   corpus albicans

   corpus luteum

   germinal epithelium

   graafin follicle

   granulosa cells

   primary follicle

   primordial follicle

   secondary follicle

   stroma

   theca externa

   theca interna

   tunica albuginea

   zona pellucida

2. In the spaces provided, draw and label pictures of the follicles at each of the different stages.

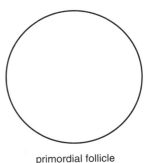

primordial follicle

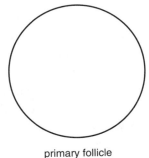

primary follicle

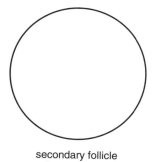

secondary follicle

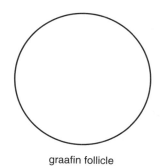

graafin follicle

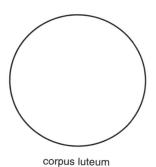

corpus luteum

Histology of the Fallopian Tube

1. Identify the following structures on the slides of the fallopian tube:

   ciliated cells

   mucosa

   muscularis

   secretory cells

   serosa

Histology of the Uterus

1. Identify the following structures on the slides of the uterus:

   endometrium

   myometrium

   perimetrium

   stratum basale

   stratum functionalis

LABORATORY REPORT QUESTIONS

Multiple Choice

Circle the letter of the correct answer.

1. As they mature, primordial follicles become _____.

   a. stroma
   b. primary follicles
   c. secondary follicle
   d. corpus luteum

2. The fluid-filled pocket within the secondary follicle is the _____.

   a. antrum
   b. corpus albicans
   c. germinal epithelium
   d. oocyte

3. The smooth muscle layer of the uterus is the _____.

   a. endometrium
   b. myometrium
   c. stroma
   d. germinal epithelium

4. After ovulation, the mature follicle regresses to become a _____.

   a. secondary follicle
   b. corpus luteum
   c. primary follicle
   d. stroma

5. The outer layer of the follicle is the _____.

   a. theca externa
   b. secretory cell layer
   c. theca interna
   d. tunica albuginea

Matching

Match the descriptions in Column A with the structures in Column B.

Column A	Column B
___ 1. Three layers of smooth muscle responsible for uterine contractions	a. stratum functionalis
___ 2. Composed of ciliated cells that transport the egg and secretory cells responsible for activating the sperm	b. granulosa cells
___ 3. Responsible for secreting the follicular fluid and estrogen in the secondary follicles	c. perimetrium
___ 4. Outermost layer of the uterus	d. myometrium
___ 5. Endometrial layer that is shed during menstruation	e. mucosa

Long Answer

1. What differentiates the primary follicle from the secondary follicle?

2. How is the corpus luteum different from the graafin follicle?

3. What is the function of the fallopian mucosa?

4. What is the role of the corpus luteum?

5. What is the zona pellucida?

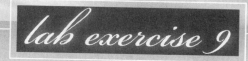

BREAST HEALTH

OBJECTIVES

At the completion of this exercise, the student should be able to:

- Identify the anatomy of the breast
- Describe the risk factors for breast cancer
- Identify the methods of breast cancer screening
- Explain the benefits and limitations of breast self-exam (BSE)
- Describe the benefits of mammography for early detection of breast cancer

MATERIALS

anatomical breast models
silicon BSE breast models (with and without tumors)

INTRODUCTION

The presence of mammary glands is one of the defining features of the animal class Mammalia. Mammals evolved the ability to secrete milk to feed their offspring in a process called lactation. In humans, mammary glands are more commonly called breasts. Both females and males have mammary tissues concentrated beneath the nipples. Before puberty, these tissues constitute the breast buds. At puberty, cells in the breast buds in girls respond to increasing estrogen levels and begin to develop. Adipose tissues deposit around the mammary tissues, the glands enlarge, and the breasts assume a more mature appearance.

BREAST STRUCTURE

The mammary tissue consists of the lactiferous ducts and the lactiferous glands, which manufacture and secrete milk. The breasts respond to the monthly hormone fluctuations associated with the menstrual cycle. Adipose and duct tissues respond especially strongly to estrogen, while progesterone has a greater effect on the lactiferous glands. The breast tenderness many women experience before their menstrual period is often due to the growth of the mammary glands in response to the progesterone peak that occurs during the third week of the menstrual cycle.

Identifing Breast Structures

Identify the following structures in Figure 9-1. After identifying the structures in Figure 9-1, locate and identify the structures on an anatomical breast model.

> adipose tissues
>
> areola
>
> lactiferous ducts
>
> lactiferous lobes and lobules
>
> ligaments
>
> nipple
>
> pectoral muscle

BREAST CANCER

Breast cancer affects one out of seven women, and is a major cause of mortality in women. Many factors contribute to a woman's risk of developing breast cancer. A family history of the disease is found in only 10 percent of breast cancers. Other contributory factors include:

- Age—breast cancer is rare before the age of 15. The frequency of breast cancer increases with age, dramatically so after menopause.

- Gender—men do develop breast cancer, but not as frequently as women do. Since breast cells respond primarily to estrogen and progesterone rather than to testosterone, women are at much greater risk.

- Late menopause—the longer a woman experiences menstrual cycles, the greater her risk of breast cancer. Both early onset of menarche and late menopause are associated with a greater risk of breast cancer.

- Childbirth and lactation—delivering and nursing a baby can decrease a woman's risk of developing breast cancer, while never having a baby increases the risk. The younger a woman is when she has her first baby and

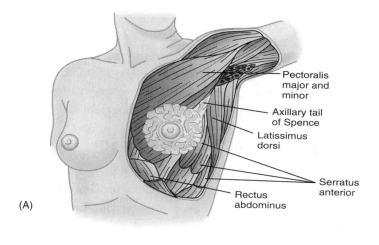

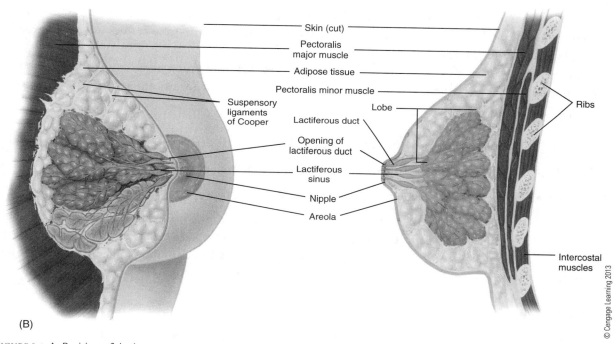

FIGURE 9-1: A. Position of the breasts in relation to the thoracic muscles. B. The internal structures of the breast.

the more children she has, the smaller her risk. However, a first delivery after age 35 can increase the risk of breast cancer. It should be noted that miscarriage and abortion have no effect, either positive or negative, on a woman's chance of developing breast cancer.

- Hormone replacement therapy (HRT)—recent research about the effects of hormone replacement therapy has shown that it significantly increases the risk of breast cancer in some postmenopausal women.

- Obesity—excess body fat and consuming high levels of dietary saturated fat are both linked to an increased risk of breast cancer. Adipose cells convert the hormone androsterendione into estrogen.

- Genetics—women who carry a mutation on the BRCA-1 and BRCA-2 genes have an increased risk of developing breast cancer. Other genetic indicators include ethnic ancestry. Women of Native American descent are at very low risk, while women of Parsi descent are at much higher risk, as are women of Northern European descent. Cultural and behavioral characteristics may also play a role.

BREAST CANCER SCREENING

Early detection is crucial to surviving breast cancer because left untreated, the cancer can metastasize to other parts of the body where it is harder to treat. Three primary methods are currently used to screen for breast cancer: breast self-examination (BSE), clinical breast exam, and mammography. Other screening methods are being developed or are currently being used to confirm the results of mammography.

Breast Self-Exam (BSE) and Clinical Breast Exam

Breast self-examination (BSE) and clinical breast exams are both manual examinations of the breasts. They rely on the sense of touch to detect abnormalities as the breasts are palpitated. The difference between the two is that a clinical breast exam is conducted by a trained healthcare professional in a clinical setting. A drawback of using BSE or clinical breast exam for early detection is that such procedures are not sensitive enough to find tumors while they are still in earliest stages. However, for women who do not have access to regular mammograms or for women who are too young to benefit from regular mammograms, clinical breast exams and self-exams may be the only screening method available. In addition, breast cancer can cause symptoms besides tumors that can be detected visually during a manual breast exam.

The textbook *Biology of Women,* 5th Edition provides detailed instructions about how to conduct breast self-examination. Conduct a breast self-exam in the privacy of your home and answer the following questions.

BSE Questions

1. Did you detect anything unusual while conducting BSE?

2. Were both breasts symmetrical or asymmetrical in terms of size, shape, and lumpiness?

3. What would be an easy way for you to incorporate BSE into your regular self-care routine?

Please note: Because of their glandular structure, most breasts feel lumpy when palpitated during a self-exam. Many women are surprised about the texture of their breasts when they first do a breast self-exam. It is important for you to know which lumps or thickenings are normal for your breasts. By becoming familiar with your existing bumps and lumps, you are more likely to notice suspicious changes if they occur.

Mammography

A mammogram is an X-ray of a breast. The American Cancer Society recommends that women have a baseline mammogram at age 40 and regular mammograms yearly or every other year thereafter. A woman's individual risk factors may dictate an earlier start to mammograms. Health insurance usually covers mammograms, but programs that provide low-cost mammograms to those without insurance coverage exist in many communities.

The advantage of mammography is that it can detect tumors that are too small to be detected by clinical breast exams or self-exams, which means that earlier-stage tumors can be identified and treated. A breast tumor of any size has the potential to metastasize and move to other parts of the body. However, tumors that are two centimeters in diameter or smaller are usually localized in the breast tissue and are easier to treat. Tumors ranging from two to five centimeters in diameter or larger are more likely to invade the lymph nodes and other tissues.

Working in small groups, students can palpitate the silicon BSE breast models to detect tumors. Interchange tumor sizes and locations to determine how effective palpitation is for detecting tumors in the breast models. Students can classify the tumor models as detectable or undetectable. Measure the detectable and undetectable tumor models to determine the average size of tumors in each category.

Silicon BSE Model Questions

1. Did the detectable and undetectable tumor models differ in size? If so, how?

2. Were most of the tumors in the detectable category likely to have been invasive or localized? Were most of the tumors in the undetectable category likely to have been invasive or localized?

3. What role does mammography play in the early detection and treatment of breast cancer?

LABORATORY REPORT QUESTIONS

Multiple Choice

Circle the letter of the correct answer.

1. Which of these is a method to detect breast cancer?
   a. mammography
   b. breast self-exam
   c. clinical breast exam
   d. all of the above

2. Breasts develop during puberty under the influence of _____.
   a. estrogen
   b. progesterone
   c. testosterone
   d. all of the above

3. The following are risk factors for breast cancer except _____.
   a. age
   b. gender
   c. family history of breast cancer
   d. history of abortion

4. The BRCA1 and BRCA2 genes_____.
   a. protect women from breast cancer
   b. are used to treat breast cancer
   c. are risk factors for developing breast cancer
   d. influence breast size

5. Mammary tissues present before puberty are called _____.
   a. areola
   b. ligaments
   c. adipose tissue
   d. breast buds

Matching

Match the descriptions in Column A with the structures in Column B.

Column A

_____ 1. Fat cells that give the breasts shape and increase their size

_____ 2. Area of darkened skin surrounding the nipple

_____ 3. Connective tissues that maintain the positions of the breasts

_____ 4. Milk flows through these to the nipple

_____ 5. Milk is manufactured here

Column B

a. lactiferous duct

b. lactiferous nodule

c. areola

d. ligaments

e. adipose tissues

Long Answer

1. What are the potential advantages and disadvantages of breast self-exam?

2. Why is the mammogram currently the preferred method for early detection of breast cancer?

3. What are the current recommendations for scheduling mammograms?

4. What role do genetics and family history play in a woman's risk of developing breast cancer?

5. Why is early detection critical to surviving breast cancer?

HEALTH AND WELLNESS PLANNER

At the completion of this exercise, the student should be able to:

- Conduct research into health information
- Evaluate health information as it relates to personal health
- Develop health and wellness goals that can be used for personal reference

internet
periodicals
publications

INTRODUCTION TO THE HEALTH AND WELLNESS PLANNER

This lab exercise involves researching health and wellness information rather than conducting a hands-on laboratory activity. Use the Internet, periodicals, and publications to gather information to develop a personal plan for health. As you research each question in the planner, you are likely to find conflicting information. Evaluate each question for yourself and fill in the best answer as it applies to you.

HEALTH AND WELLNESS PLANNER

Personal Research and Brainstorming

Research the answers to each of the following questions, making sure to carefully document original sources.

1a. How much exercise should I get per day? Per week?

1b. Which kinds of exercise should I be getting and how much of each (i.e, aerobic, strength, stretching)?

1d. Which activities can I include in my day/week during each of the four seasons to make sure I get enough exercise?

2a. How many calories should I consume per day?

2b. How many grams of protein should I consume per day? What does this look like in servings?

2c. How many grams of carbohydrate should I consume per day? What does this look like in servings?

2d. How many grams of fat should I consume per day? How many servings is this?

2e. How many grams of fiber should I consume per day? Examples of the foods I need to include in a typical day to get my daily recommendation of fiber include:

3. Should I be taking vitamin or mineral supplements? If so, what dosages would be optimal?

4a. How many hours of sleep should I get per night? What are the benefits of getting the recommended amount of sleep?

4b. Do I need to modify my daily schedule to get more or less sleep? If so, how can I adjust my schedule?

5. What am I currently doing to improve or enhance my emotional/mental health? What activities or habits would I like to adopt to improve or enhance my emotional/mental health?

6a. What is my risk level for the following health conditions (a simple evaluation of low, medium, or high risk is sufficient)?

   a. heart disease

   b. osteoporosis

   c. cancer (breast, cervical, colon, lung, etc.)

   d. diabetes

   e. stress and/or depression

   f. eating disorders

   g. perimenopause or menopause (for male students, prostate problems)

   h. arthritis

   i. addictions

   j. other

6b. I am at medium to high risk for:

6c. What specific things can I do to improve my chances of remaining healthy or improving my current health with respect to my risk areas? (Use a separate sheet of paper if necessary.)

6d. Which medical tests or screenings, if any, should I schedule this year?

Goal Setting

My physical fitness goals for the upcoming year:

a.

b.

My emotional/mental health goals for the upcoming year:

a.

b.

My general health goals for the upcoming year:

a.

b.

Measuring Progress

Your progress can be measured in many ways, depending on what is important to you! For example, you can measure your physical fitness progress by looking at changes in blood pressure, flexibility, cholesterol, strength, energy level, improved sense of well-being, or weight and inches gained or lost. Use more than one criterion to measure your progress. How will you measure your progress for your physical fitness, emotional/mental health, and general health goals?

Physical Fitness Goals:

a.

b.

Emotional/Mental Health Goals:

a.

b.

General Health Goals:

a.

b.

LABORATORY REPORT QUESTIONS

Long Answer

1. Reflect on your answers to Question 1. Were there any surprises?

2. Reflect on your answers to questions 2-4. Did you learn anything in your research that will influence your daily choices?

3. What did you learn about yourself while researching answers to the questions in the Health and Wellness Planner?

4. Which Web resource or other resource did you find most helpful? Why?

FITNESS LAB—MEASURING YOUR FITNESS LEVEL

At the completion of this exercise, the student should be able to:

- Identify the components that contribute to fitness
- Explain why a single measure of fitness does not present a full picture
- Identify a personal level of fitness

8-pound weight
ruler
scale
stopwatch
tape measure
two thick books
weight/height charts

INTRODUCTION

Over time, the standards of fitness have changed. In an attempt to measure fitness, the insurance industry developed height and weight charts to use as a basis for assessing risk when insuring prospective policyholders. In theory, people above the "acceptable" weight for their height were considered in poor health and, therefore, were regarded as an insurance risk. In recent years, body mass index, or BMI, has become a standard method for measuring fitness. BMI is useful but does not take into account that lean muscle weighs more than fat. An athlete will have a higher BMI than a person of the same body size who does not exercise. Both height/weight charts and BMI measurements focus on weight as the measure of fitness, excluding other factors.

More recent fitness assessments consider a variety of factors, rather than a single one, when calculating fitness. These measures usually include a combination of flexibility, strength, and endurance or aerobic capacity. Flexibility is a measure of the range of movement of tendons, ligaments, and muscles. Increased flexibility increases the range of motion in joints. A loss of flexibility is often associated with aging and injury. Strength is a measure of how much force muscles can exert. Because different muscle groups are used to differing extents, one muscle group may be quite strong while another is much weaker. For example, women typically have strong leg muscles but often lack upper body strength. Training can improve the strength of muscles, encourage osteoblast activity, and limit the effects of osteoporosis. Endurance is a measure of a muscle's ability to sustain activity and aerobic capacity. Aerobic capacity is a measure of the heart and lung's ability to deliver oxygen to the muscles. Without adequate oxygen, muscles tire quickly. In response to demands for oxygen by the muscles, the heart and respiratory rates increase. How quickly the heart rate returns to a resting rate is a measure of aerobic capacity. Like strength, endurance can be improved through training.

PROCEDURES

In this lab exercise, you will take an initial evaluation of your fitness level. From that information, you will identify an aspect of your fitness that you feel you can improve. Over the course of the semester, you will incorporate physical activities to improve the area you identified. Finally, at the end of the semester, you will repeat the fitness assessment for comparison.

If you have limitations that make any of these activities hazardous for you, consult your instructor.

BMI and Weight/Height Measures

1. Measure your weight and height, recording the values.

2. Using the height/weight chart provided, identify if you are below, above, or at your optimal weight.

3. Calculate your BMI:

    weight in pounds _____ × 0.45 = _____ kg

    height in inches _____ × 0.0254 = _____ meters

    $$BMI = \frac{\text{weight in kg}}{(\text{height in meters})^2} = \underline{\hspace{2cm}}$$

BMI below 20 = underweight

20–25 = normal

25–30 = overweight

over 30 = obese

Flexibility Assessment 1

1. Stand barefoot with your feet together and your knees relaxed.

2. Reach for the floor.

3. Rate your ability to touch the floor.

   No contact = 0 points

   Fingertips = 1 point

   Fist = 2 points

   Palms = 3 points

4. Record the points on the report form.

Flexibility Assessment 2

1. Stack two books, one atop the other.

2. Sit on the floor with your legs in front of you.

3. With your feet flat against the books and bending from the hips, use your fingers to slowly push the top book as far forward as possible.

4. Measure the distance you were able to push the top book.

   0–1 inch = 1 point

   1–2 inches = 2 points

   2–3 inches = 3 points

   3–4 inches = 4 points

   More than 4 inches = 5 points

5. Record the points on the report form.

Strength Assessment

1. Using the 8-pound weight, perform arm curls with your right arm.

2. Stop when your arm tires.

3. Record the points based on the number of right arm curls.

   Fewer than 20 arm curls = 1 point

   21–40 arm curls = 2 points

   41–60 arm curls = 3 points

4. Repeat the process with the left arm and record the results.

Aerobic capacity

1. Take your pulse before beginning to walk.

   Resting pulse _____

2. Walk for five minutes at a moderate pace. You want to be able to carry on a conversation.

3. When you finish the walk, take your pulse again.

   End pulse _____

4. Take your pulse every minute until it returns to your resting rate.

   _____ minutes to return to the resting rate

5. Record the points on the report form.

   > 1 minute or less = 4 points
   >
   > 2–4 minutes = 3 points
   >
   > 5–7 minutes = 2 points
   >
   > More than 7 minutes = 1 point

LAB REPORT FORM

	Initial Assessment	Final Assessment
Height		
Weight		
Measure by height/weight chart		
BMI		

1. Do the results from the height/weight chart agree with the BMI results?

	Initial Assessment Points	Final Assessment Points
Flexibility 1		
Flexibility 2		
Right Arm Curls		
Left Arm Curls		
Aerobic Capacity		
Point Totals		

Overall Fitness Scores

15–18 points = excellent

11–14 points = good

7–10 points = average

Fewer than 7 points = below average

1. Did you find areas in which you were especially strong? Did you find areas in which you were especially weak?

2. When doing the arm curls, did you see a difference between the right arm and the left arm?

3. Based on these results, identify an area to improve.

4. What changes will you make to your lifestyle to improve in this area?

5. Did you continue the activity between the initial and final assessments?

6. Did you find changes in your results between the initial and final assessment?

LABORATORY REPORT QUESTIONS

Multiple Choice

Circle the letter of the correct answer.

1. Body mass indexing _____.
   a. measures aerobic capacity
   b. relates height to weight
   c. increases with training
   d. measure joint mobility

2. _____ has the potential to reduce the effects of osteoporosis.
   a. A reduced BMI
   b. Reducing aerobic capacity
   c. Reducing endurance
   d. Strength training

3. The ability to touch the floor while standing is a measure of _____.
   a. strength
   b. flexibility
   c. weight/height
   d. aerobic capacity

4. Increasing oxygen delivery to the muscles will improve _____.

   a. strength
   b. flexibility
   c. the height/weight ratio
   d. endurance

5. The units of BMI are _____.

   a. inch^2/meter
   b. kilogram/meter^2
   c. pounds/inch^2
   d. kilogram/pound

Matching

Match the descriptions in Column A with the concepts in Column B.

Column A

____ 1. A measure of oxygen delivery and usage by muscles

____ 2. Mathematical relationship between weight and height

____ 3. Amount of force exerted by a muscle

____ 4. Amount of movement in tendons and ligaments

____ 5. Method for improving fitness

Column B

a. strength

b. flexibility

c. training

d. aerobic capacity

e. BMI

Long Answer

1. Why is a single test an inadequate measure of fitness?

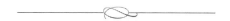

2. Explain why one muscle group can be strong and another weak in the same individual.

3. Why can two people with identical height and shape have two different BMIs?

4. How does oxygen delivery relate to endurance?

5. What kind of activities can increase aerobic capacity?

STRESS REDUCTION LAB

OBJECTIVES

At the completion of this exercise, the student should be able to:

- Describe the effects of stress on the body
- Describe several methods for reducing the effects of stress on the body
- Identify one or more techniques that work for the individual student

MATERIALS

chocolate
lavender aromatherapy candles
relaxation CD or DVD
yoga mat or blanket

INTRODUCTION

Whether in one's personal life, school, or work, stress affects everyone at some point. The stress response can be triggered by both positive events, such as a new job or the birth of a child, or negative situations, such as a car accident or an unpleasant boss. Both types of situations will provoke a similar response by the body. The stress response can have a number of negative effects on the body, including:

- activation of the sympathetic nervous system (the "fight-or-flight" response)
- increased adrenalin secretion, which
  - increases heart rate
  - increases respiratory rate
  - increases blood pressure
- increased cortisol levels, which
  - depress the immune system
  - increase blood sugar levels
  - increase the breakdown of skin fat
- increased LDL (low density lipoprotein) levels
- increased storage of abdominal fat

In addition to the physiological changes, stress can trigger sleepless nights, an inability to concentrate, and changes in behavior. Chronic stress is associated with weight gain, heart disease, cancer, diabetes, autoimmune conditions, asthma, and depression. Lowering stress reduces these negative effects on the body, and people have developed a number of methods for handling stress.

This lab exercise is designed to allow you to explore several stress-reduction methods in class and at home, and to identify those that work best for you. To evaluate the success of each method, you will look at your pulse rate before and after each stress-reduction activity. This is a quantitative measure, and the pulse rate before the stress-reduction activity acts as the baseline. A reduction in the pulse rate indicates activation of the parasympathetic nervous system and relaxation. Some activities may not produce a change in pulse rate but may make you feel more relaxed. How you feel after each activity is a subjective, qualitative measure; yet, it is still a measure of stress reduction. Finally, you will determine how viable the option is for you. Not all stress-reduction methods can be used at all times. For example, taking 15 minutes for a quick massage in the middle of an exam or practicing yoga while driving in a traffic jam are not necessarily viable options. Other methods such as deep breathing can be practiced anywhere. By testing several methods, you can gather a collection of stress-reduction techniques that you can draw upon as the situation warrants.

STRESS-REDUCTION OPTIONS

The following is a representative collection of stress-reduction ideas and explanations as to why they work. This is not an exhaustive list, just examples generally recognized as useful for coping with stress. Your instructor may assign other options for you to try.

- Deep breathing—As trivial as it sounds, deep breathing can be highly effective for relieving stress. One of our first responses to pain is to hold our breath, and we do the same thing when we are stressed. Shallow breathing decreases the oxygen supply to our muscles and brain. This, in turn, decreases their function and alters the metabolism. Try just taking five or six deep breaths. Breathe in on a count of 3, hold for a count of 3, and exhale on a count of 3.

- Exercise—Whether it is a walk outside or a full hour of kickboxing, exercise is well recognized as a stress reducer. When you exercise, you breathe more deeply. You also produce endorphins – natural opiate compounds that have a calming effect on the nervous system. Exercise also shifts your focus, literately taking your mind off your problems, if only for a little while. For evaluation purposes, wait at least 20 minutes before taking your pulse.

- Aromatherapy—Studies have shown that certain scents alter brain chemistry. Aromas trigger some of the deepest, most subconscious parts of the brain. If a specific smell has positive associations for you, use it. A number of odors are documented as associated with physiological responses. For example, peppermint sharpens brain functioning; lavender and hops have soothing effects. Sandalwood, rosemary, and frankincense are recognized bronchodilators (they open up the lungs to increase air flow) and help people to relax.

- Shower or bath—For most people, water is soothing. A long soak in a warm bathtub can soothe away many stresses. Add a little aromatherapy, a few candles, shut off the phone, and relax. The warm water dilates the blood vessels at the skin surface (increasing oxygen delivery and lowering blood pressure) and the heat loosens tight muscles.

- Meditation—As a stress reliever, meditation has been shown to lower the heart rate, decrease blood pressure, and lower anxiety by altering brain chemistry. Many meditation CDs are available for sale, and your local public library may also have several in its CD collection. Then, set aside some undisturbed time to listen and relax.

- Laughter—When you laugh, the brain releases endorphins. Try a funny movie, a TV comedy, going out with friends, or playing with puppies.

- A good book—Create a personal ritual of reading something neither school or work related for 10 to 15 minutes a day. Grab a romance, mystery, fantasy, a classic—anything you don't have to read for a class. Reading for pleasure can help you relax.

- Chocolate—In most cases, using food as a coping mechanism is not a healthy choice, but chocolate may be an exception. The feel of chocolate in the mouth triggers the parasympathetic system and reduces stress. Chemicals in chocolate mimic neurotransmitters associated with a sense of well-being. Chocolate also contains many of the essential trace minerals. While it is not a good idea to eat a whole pound of chocolate, savoring a few bites of really good chocolate can be an effective way to reduce stress.

- Yoga—Many people find yoga soothing. It stretches muscles, loosens joints, and helps you focus on your breathing. Most libraries have yoga DVDs, and yoga classes are offered by many community organizations.

- Massage—Touch releases a whole set of chemicals in the brain. For most people, these are associated with feelings of safety and comfort. Massage increases circulation and loosens tight muscles. It can also be used to help you identify those areas in which you carry your stress, allowing you to consciously work on relaxing those muscles.

- Find a hobby—Engage in pleasurable activities—gardening, crafts, dance, music—any activity that lets you escape from your everyday routine. For many people in today's society, creativity is suppressed; that in itself can create stress. Hobbies typically activate different areas of the brain and can be very soothing.

STRESS-REDUCTION LAB REPORT FORM

Try four stress-reducing options from the list above. After each activity:

- Record your pulse before and after.

- Consider how you feel after the activity. Is the activity a viable option to help you reduce stress? Why or why not?

Option	Pulse before	Pulse after	How do you feel?	Did activity reduce your heart rate?

© Cengage Learning 2013

1. Which method is most effective for you?

2. Were any of the methods not relaxing for you?

3. Compare your results with those of others in your class. Did you respond the same way to the stress-reduction techniques?

LABORATORY REPORT QUESTIONS

Multiple Choice

Circle the letter of the correct answer.

1. In response to a stressful situation, the body normally _____.

    a. decreases the heart rate
    b. triggers the sympathetic nervous system
    c. decreases cortisol levels
    d. activates the parasympathetic nervous system

2. Elevated levels of cortisol _____.

    a. activate the parasympathetic nervous system
    b. decrease blood sugar levels
    c. increase fat storage in the skin
    d. reduce immune system function

3. Asthma, autoimmune conditions, and depression are linked to _____.

    a. chronic stress
    b. increased exercise
    c. decreased LDL levels
    d. relaxation

4. Controlled, deep breathing helps the body counter the effects of stress by _____.

    a. reducing neurotransmitter levels
    b. lowering LDL levels
    c. increasing the heart rate
    d. increasing oxygen delivery to the brain

Matching

Match the description in Column A with the stress-reduction method in Column B.

Column A

____ 1. Dilates blood vessels in the skin, relaxes muscles, lowers blood pressure

____ 2. Increases blood flow, increases the respiratory rate, increases the heart rate

____ 3. Stretches muscles, improves joint flexibility, helps control breathing

____ 4. Dilates the bronchioles in the lung

____ 5. Increases brain activity

Column B

a. frankincense

b. peppermint

c. exercise

d. yoga

e. bath

Long Answer

1. Why is chronic stress damaging to the body?

2. How can you quickly tell if you are relaxing?

3. In popular media, characters under stress often eat chocolate. Why might this actually work to make the character feel better?

4. How does exercise help to reduce the stress response?

5. Are there other techniques that help you, personally, relax?

SEXUALLY TRANSMITTED INFECTIONS LAB

OBJECTIVES

At the completion of this exercise, the student will be able to:

- Identify select organisms that cause sexually transmitted infections (STIs)
- Describe the symptoms of select STIs
- Describe the STI treatments available
- Explain how to prevent the transmission of STIs

MATERIALS

brochures and reference materials on STIs
immersion oil
lens paper
microscope
prepared microscope slides of each of the following:

    Chlamydia trachomatis
    Neisseria gonorrhea
    Phthirus pubis
    Treponema pallidum
    Trichomonas vaginalis

INTRODUCTION

Anyone who is sexually active needs to be concerned about sexually transmitted infections (STIs). STIs are infections most often passed between sexual partners through intimate contact. Semen and vaginal secretions may contain organisms, even in those who show no symptoms of the infection. These microscopic organisms can be passed through skin-to-skin contact or through contact with the blood of an infected person. Many STIs are capable of crossing the placenta and attacking a fetus as it develops. Other pathogens can be transmitted to a baby during delivery. Limiting transmission of the microbes is one of the most effective methods of controlling sexually transmitted infections.

The sexually transmitted infection known as syphilis is cause by the bacterium *Treponema pallidum* (Figure 13-1). This organism is a minute spiral that stains red with a gram stain. During the primary stage of the infection, the lesions produced at the point the organism enters the body create highly infectious fluids teeming with bacteria. However, the lesion is often overlooked, and the infection can move into the bloodstream if left untreated. During the secondary stages of the infection, the bacteria can also be found in the blood.

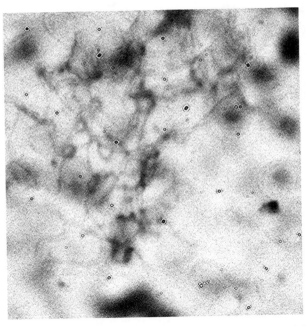

FIGURE 13-1: *Treponema pallidum.* (Courtesy of Theresa Hornstein)

The infection known as gonorrhea is caused by the bacterium *Neisseria gonorrhea* (Figure 13-2). Women infected with gonorrhea often exhibit no symptoms. However, in men classic symptoms include painful urination and a pus discharge from the penis. The bacterial organism destroys cells lining both the vas deferens and the fallopian tubes, producing scarring that can lead to infertility. In a prepared slide, the bacteria appear as pairs of spheres that stain red in a gram stain.

Chlamydia trachomatis is an intracellular parasite which lives in the cells of the reproductive system. Infections are often asymptomatic in both men and women. However, the organism can produce scarring of the reproductive tract leading to infertility. The organism can be passed to newborns during a vaginal delivery, leading to pneumonia and eye infections if left untreated. In a prepared slide, the organism appears as round cells often within the human cells.

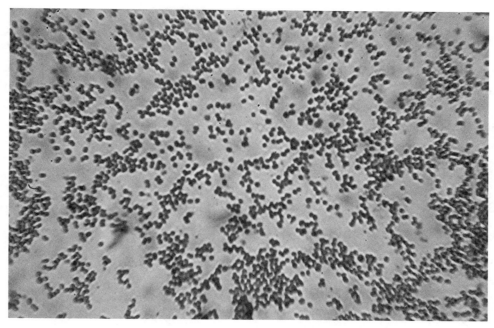

FIGURE 13-2: *Neisseria gonorrhea* (Courtesy of CDC/Dr. Stuart Brown)

Trichomonas vaginalis (Figure 13-3) is a flagellated protozoan. This organism can cause an unpleasant odor and frothy vaginal discharge in women. Men infected with trichomonas usually exhibit no symptoms, but can pass the organism to their partners.

Phthirus pubis is the pubic louse. This six-legged insect attaches to the pubic hair and feeds off the host's blood. An infestation produces itching and small lesions at the site of the bites. The organism is passed through close contact including sexual activity and shared clothing.

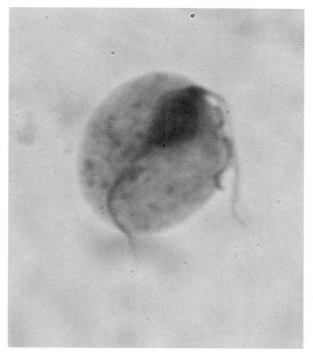

FIGURE 13-3: *Trichomonas vaginalis.* (Courtesy of Theresa Hornstein)

Identifying a sexually transmitted infection depends on symptoms and lab results. Laboratory testing can identify such infections before symptoms appear. Many of the organisms that cause STIs are too small to be seen with the naked eye, making microscopic examination one method of identifying the organisms. Understanding which organisms can cause STIs, how an STI is transmitted, and symptoms of an STI can reduce an individual's risk of becoming infected. The Centers for Disease Control (www.cdc.gov), the World Health Organization (www.who.int), and the National Women's Health Information Center (www.womenshealth.gov) provide detailed and accurate information concerning STIs.

PROCEDURES

Microscopic Examination of Select Organisms

1. Using oil immersion, examine prepared slides of the following organisms.

2. Sketch pictures of the organisms in the spaces provided.

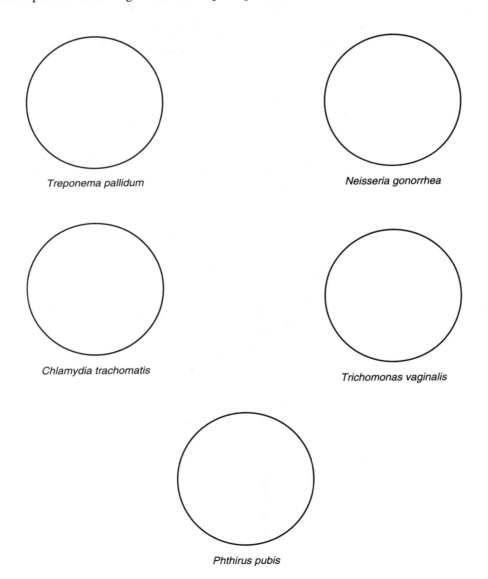

Treponema pallidum

Neisseria gonorrhea

Chlamydia trachomatis

Trichomonas vaginalis

Phthirus pubis

Symptoms, Prevention, and Treatment Options

1. Using all the resources available to you, complete the following chart:

	Description of organism	List of symptoms	How to prevent transmission	Treatment
Chlamydia trachomatis				
hepatitis B (HBV)				
herpes simplex				
human immunodeficiency virus (HIV)				
human papilloma virus (HPV)				
Neisseria gonorrhea				
Phthirus pubis				
Treponema pallidum				
Trichomonas vaginalis				

LABORATORY REPORT QUESTIONS

Multiple Choice

Circle the letter of the correct answer.

1. *Phthirus pubis* are _____.

   a. public lice
   b. bacteria
   c. protozoans
   d. viruses

2. Which STI can be prevented by vaccination?

   a. HIV
   b. herpes simplex
   c. *Treponema pallidum*
   d. HPV

3. Which of the following can be treated with antibiotics?

   a. HPV
   b. herpes simplex
   c. *Chlamydia trachomatis*
   d. *Phthirus pubis*

4. _____ use flagella to move through the reproductive tract.

   a. *Trichamonas vaginalis*
   b. HPV
   c. *Chlamydia trachomatis*
   d. *Neisseria gonorrhea*

5. The small spiral bacterium that causes syphilis is _____.

   a. *Neisseria gonorrhea*
   b. HIV
   c. HBV
   d. *Treponema pallidum*

Matching

Match the symptoms in Column A with the organisms in Column B.

Column A	Column B
C 1. liver failure, jaundice, fever, tiredness, loss of appetite	a. herpes simplex
b 2. small painless lesions, muscle aches, a rash on palms and soles that does not itch	b. *Treponema pallidum*
e 3. foamy vaginal discharge with a strong odor, genital itching	c. HIV
C 4. recurrent painful, weeping blisters; muscle aches; pain in genital area	d. HBV
d 5. fever, weight loss, diarrhea, depressed immune system	e. *Trichomonas vaginalis*

Long Answer

1. How are STIs transmitted?

2. Why are pregnant women tested for HIV and *Treponema pallidum*?

3. Is vaginal intercourse the only way to become infected with an STI?

4. Why are condoms effective at preventing the transmission of some, but not all, STIs?

5. How can someone be infected with an STI and not know it?

BIRTH CONTROL

At the completion of this exercise, the student should be able to:

- Describe different methods of birth control and explain how they work
- Identify local sources for obtaining birth control
- Determine the best birth control method for her/his current lifestyle

informational brochures on birth control methods
samples of birth control methods

INTRODUCTION

Throughout human history—probably since the first time sexual activity was connected with pregnancy—humans have sought methods to control their fertility. In nomadic peoples, being able to time births and the last stages of pregnancy to avoid the migrations was a necessity. Deliveries while traveling posed severe risks to both mother and child. In areas where famine was seasonal, timing births to match times of plenty also improved survival rates.

Today, a range of safe and effective birth control methods exist. **Barrier methods** use a physical barrier to prevent sperm from reaching an egg. Barrier methods are more effective when combined with **chemical methods** (spermicides) which immobilize and kill sperm. IUDs are a physical method which creates an environment in the uterus which is inhospitable to an egg. **Hormonal methods** of birth control use synthetic forms of estrogen or progesterone to disrupt the reproductive cycle in women. By altering the levels of these hormones, ovulation is inhibited and the endometrial lining is altered to reduce the possibility of implantation. However, these methods are effective only when a person knows where to obtain them and how to use them. Organizations such as Planned Parenthood and the World Health Organization as well as local health care personnel can provide accurate information about birth control methods. ,including their effectiveness and safety. Some women have medical conditions that make the use of certain birth control methods unsafe. For example, hormonal forms of birth control are contraindicated—considered unsafe—for women with a history of estrogen-dependent breast cancer or cardiovascular disease. Many methods of birth control are available without prescriptions; others are available only through a health care professional. For this lab exercise, you will research several birth control methods and identify those that are available over the counter locally.

UNDERSTANDING BIRTH CONTROL METHODS

1. For each of the following birth control methods, describe how it works and any contraindications, benefits, and side effects.

Method	How it works	Contraindications	Benefits	Side effects
abstinence				
diaphragm/ cervical cap				
condom				

hormonal methods (oral contraceptives, injectable, contraceptive patch)				
IUD				
spermicide				
emergency contraception				
natural family planning				

2. Research the availability of birth control options in your community. Visit at least two stores and identify the birth control methods each provides over the counter.

3. For yourself, identify the birth control method that would best fit your current life situation.

LABORATORY REPORT QUESTIONS

Multiple Choice

Circle the letter of the correct answer.

1. Barrier methods work by _____.

   a. killing sperm
   b. preventing the sperm from contacting the egg
   c. preventing ovulation
   d. preventing sperm production

2. Hormonal birth control methods work by _____.

   a. killing sperm
   b. preventing the sperm from contacting the egg
   c. preventing ovulation
   d. preventing sperm production

3. _____ do not require a prescription or visit to a health care provider.

   a. Injectable contraceptives
   b. Birth control pills
   c. IUDs
   d. Emergency contraceptives

4. Women who smoke and are over 35 should avoid which birth control method?

   a. condoms
   b. birth control pills
   c. copper IUDs
   d. natural family planning

5. Which birth control method is used by men?

   a. injectable contraceptives
   b. birth control pills
   c. condoms
   d. cervical caps

Matching

Match the birth control method in Column A with a description of how it works in Column B.

Column A

___ 1. condom

___ 2. Depo-Provera

___ 3. emergency contraception

___ 4. spermicide

___ 5. cervical cap

Column B

a. barrier method

b. prevent ovulation

c. kills sperm

Long Answer

1. Why is it important to know where to obtain birth control?

2. What could be a contraindication to using a specific birth control method?

3. What birth control methods are available over the counter in your local stores?

PREGNANCY AND DEVELOPMENT

OBJECTIVES

At the completion of this exercise, the student should be able to:

- List the stages of development from fertilized egg to a fetus
- Describe the developmental processes that facilitate embryonic and early fetal development
- Identify the three germ layers
- Identify the cellular origins of the organ systems

MATERIALS

lens paper
microscope
prepared whitefish blastula microscope slides
prepared starfish or sea urchin development microscope slides
prepared chick development microscope slides
scientific embryo and fetus models

INTRODUCTION

After egg and sperm fuse to form a fertilized egg, all animals undergo a remarkably similar series of developmental stages as they mature. The timing of each stage varies between species. However, the processes that take place and the appearance of each of the stages of the developing embryo are frequently indistinguishable, even when comparing distantly related species. This is particularly true during the earliest stages of development. This uniformity, along with the sizeable percentage of genes that are shared, is evidence of the interrelatedness of all animals.

DEVELOPMENTAL STAGES

Because the processes that take place and the appearance of the stages are similar among animals, it is possible to use distantly related animal species as models for human development. For this lab exercise, microscope slides of whitefish, starfish, or sea urchin embryos will be used to demonstrate the early stages of embryonic development, including the early cleavage through the gastrula stage. Chick embryos will be used to examine later stages of embryonic and fetal development, including the neural tube formation and development of the body systems. Examine the corresponding microscope slides and identify the stages and structures described in the following sections.

Early Cleavage Divisions

In an unfertilized egg or primary **oocyte,** the nucleus, which appears as a dark circle within a larger circle, is readily visible under low magnification. Once fertilized, the nuclear membrane disappears and the entire egg is filled with chromatin, which will appear dark. You may be able to find cells that are in the very early stages of the merger between the egg and the sperm, in which each individual nucleus can be seen prior to its fusion (Figure 15-1). The fertilized egg is called a **zygote.**

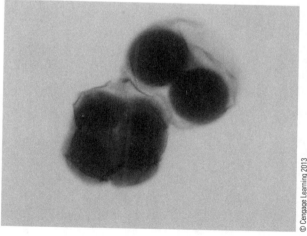

FIGURE 15-1: Early cleavages.

© Cengage Learning 2013

Following the first division, the egg appears as two cells surrounded by a fertilization membrane. This two-cell (or first cleavage) stage occupies no more space than the unfertilized egg. Each cell is referred to as a **blastomere.** The first several cleavages do not increase the size of the zygote; instead, the size of each new cell decreases as the number increases. The two-celled zygote will undergo additional cleavages to become a 4-cell, 8-cell, and then 16-cell solid ball of cells. This solid ball of cells is referred to as a **morula** (Figure 15-2). By the 16-cell stage, the cell division begins to become uneven with the formation of larger macromeres, the slightly smaller mesomeres, and tiny micromeres. You may not be able to distinguish the size differences. From this point, the cell divisions become more and more uneven.

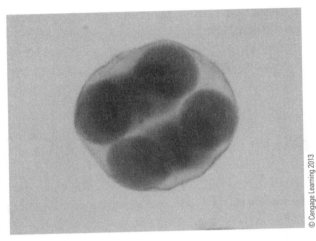

FIGURE 15-2: Morula.

Blastula Stage

The formation of the **blastula** signals the end of the cleavage stages. The blastula appears as a hollow ball of tiny embryonic cells surrounding an empty cavity (Figure 15-3). The cavity is called the **blastocoel.** The blastocoel will begin to fill with new cells along one edge, causing one wall of the blastula to become several layers thick. This inner cell layer will eventually form the embryo. The outer layer of cells is called the **trophoblast,** and in humans, it will become part of the placenta and the fetal membranes.

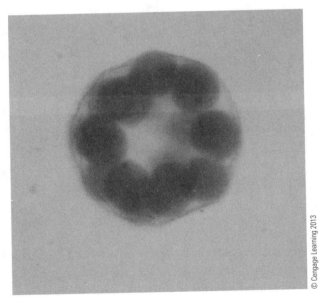

FIGURE 15-3: Blastocyst.

Gastrula Stage

Gastrulation is the formation of a three-layered embryo. In humans, gastrulation takes place after the blastula burrows into the endoderm of the uterus, and is therefore difficult to see. In starfish and sea urchins, however, gastrulation is easy to observe. The uneven rate of cell division described earlier allows the inner cell mass to grow very rapidly and fold over and into the blastocoel, eventually squeezing it out of existence. The folding produces three layers of tissue: the endoderm, mesoderm, and ectoderm. These layers are called germ layers, and each gives rise to distinct organs and tissues in the body. The outer layer, the **ectoderm,** will become the integumentary system and the nervous system. The middle layer, the **mesoderm,** forms the muscles, skeleton, and many of the internal organs. The inner layer, the **endoderm,** forms the major endocrine glands, linings of the respiratory and digestive tracts, the bladder, and stem cells that will eventually form gametes. After gastrulation, the gastrula is called an **embryo.** The embryo will begin to lengthen at this point and further development will progress from the "head" end toward the tail end.

Development of the Neural Groove

In animals that have a backbone, the brain and spinal cord are the next structures to develop. After gastrualtion, a fold becomes visible toward the head end of the embryo. Neural crests, which are ridges of ectoderm, begin to fold upward and merge to form a structure called the neural tube. This tube will become the brain and spinal cord. Below the neural tube, a dense group of cells called the notochord can sometimes be observed. These cells will contribute to the formation of the vertebra.

Development of Body Systems

In the 26- to 29-hour chick embryo slides, a number of details become visible. The neural groove is sealing from the head toward the tail. Beside the neural groove are the somites, which appear as small blocks of dense tissue. The somites will develop into several body organs. In the 40- to 45-hour chick embryo, the heart has begun to form, optic discs are visible, and the brain has begun to differentiate. A large network of blood vessels can be seen radiating from the embryo. In the human embryo, organ development will continue until the ninth week of gestation. At this stage, the embryo becomes a fetus. During the remaining weeks of the pregnancy, the organ systems continue to develop and the fetus grows larger.

LABORATORY REPORT QUESTIONS

Multiple Choice

Circle the letter of the correct answer.

1. The fertilized egg is called a(n) _____.
   - a. embryo
   - b. blastula
   - c. fetus
   - d. zygote

2. The three germ layers form during the _____.
   - a. blastula stage
   - b. neural groove formation
   - c. gastrulation
   - d. fetal stage

3. The neural tube will eventually become the _____.

   a. backbone
   b. brain and spinal cord
   c. skin
   d. skeleton

4. As the fertilized egg divides, it undergoes _____.

   a. gastrulation
   b. neural tube formation
   c. somite formation
   d. cleavage

5. In one development stage, a hollow ball of cells is called a(n) _____.

   a. embryo
   b. gastrula
   c. blastula
   d. zygote

Matching

Match the phrases in Column A with the structures in Column B.

Column A	Column B
____ 1. The first stage of development	a. morula
____ 2. The second stage of development	b. fetus
____ 3. The third stage of development	c. embryo
____ 4. The fourth stage of development	d. zygote
____ 5. The fifth stage of development	e. gastrula
____ 6. The sixth stage of development	f. blastula
____ 7. The seventh stage of development	g. neural tube formation

Long Answer

1. Why is it possible to observe starfish or chicken embryos to understand human development?

2. How are the endoderm, mesoderm, and ectoderm different from one another?

3. What is the role of the somites?

4. Describe how the fetal stage is different from the embryo stage.

5. Describe how a morula and and a blastula are different, and how are they similar.

6. Which organs form first during embryonic development? Why is this?

BIOLOGY OF APPEARANCE

OBJECTIVES

At the completion of this exercise, the student should be able to:

- Discuss the role of appearance in social species
- Describe the structure of the major components of the integument: the skin, hair, and fingernails
- Explain the role of melanocytes in the skin
- Describe the characteristics that influence hair texture

MATERIALS

anatomical models of skin, hair, and fingernails
microscope
prepared hair microscope slides
prepared human thick skin microscope slides
prepared melanocyte microscope slides

INTRODUCTION

Many factors influence a person's physical appearance, including skeletal structure, adipose distribution, eye color, and the color and texture of the skin and hair. Some of these factors are influenced by genetics, and others are influenced by passive environmental factors or purposeful modification. Scientists have explored many factors that contribute to the importance of appearance in social species, particularly human beings. For visual species, distinct appearance allows individual recognition and the establishment of social bonds. In many species, appearance plays a role in mate selection and can be used to estimate the reproductive capacity of a potential mate. Appearance also gives an indication of general health and genetic fitness to be passed on to the offspring.

EXAMINE SKIN UNDER THE MICROSCOPE

The skin is made up of two layers, the epidermis and the dermis. The **epidermis,** the outer layer, is made up of layers of regenerating cells that are constantly shed from the surface. The deepest layer of cells in the epiderimis consists of living cells that divide to make new cells. As the new cells are pushed toward the surface, they fill with a protein called keratin, which makes the cells tougher but also kills them by the time they reach the surface. This process of regeneration by the epidermis allows the skin to withstand abrasion and injury as it is exposed to the elements. The **dermis** consists of collagen and other connective tissues, which give the skin resilience and the ability to stretch and move as the muscles move underneath it. Blood vessels, nerves, sweat glands, and hair follicles are found in the dermis. Associated with the hair follicles are sebaceous glands, which secrete an oily substance called sebum to maintain each hair follicle. Muscles called the arrector pili attach to each hair follicle. When these contract, they cause the hairs to stand up in response to cold temperatures or alarm. In species with fur, the result is a fluffing of the fur, which can either make the animal appear larger and more fierce or provide added insulation against cold. Lacking fur, the contraction of arrector pili muscles in humans results in goose bumps.

Deep to the dermis and closely associated with the skin is the **hypodermis,** or subcutaneous layer. The hypodermis is similar in structure to the dermis except that it contains more adipose tissue. Adipose tissue provide several important functions. It provides insulation and padding to protect the body organs, and it also stores energy. Adipose tissue also contributes to an individual's shape, including the changes in the shape of the hips and breasts as females undergo puberty.

Identify the location and function of the following structures in Figure 16-1 and in the skin sample slide under the microscope.

adipose tissue

arrector pili muscle

blood vessel

dermis

epidermis

hair follicle

hypodermis

nerve

sebaceous gland

sweat gland

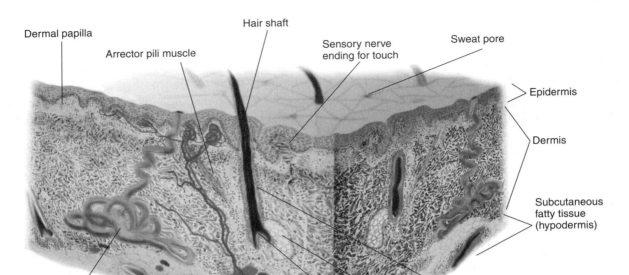

FIGURE 16-1: The structure of the skin.

MELANOCYTES

Melanocytes are cells that produce melanin, an important pigment that contributes to skin color. Melanocytes are manufactured and maintained in the epidermis. Melanin is an important component of the skin because it protects the tissues and organs below the epidermis from the damaging effects of ultraviolet radiation. All people (except albinos) have melanin in their skin. The amount varies by individual, which accounts for variations in human skin color. The baseline level of melanin in the skin and hair is determined by genetics, but melanin production can also be influenced by ultraviolet exposure. The skin manufactures additional melanin when exposed to increased sunlight, resulting in the darker skin tone of a suntan.

Examine the microscope slide showing melanocytes. Where are melanocytes located in the skin? Why is this location important?

HAIR FOLLICLES

Individual hairs are made up of concentric layers of connective tissue, primarily a protein called **keratin.** The center of the hair shaft is called the **medulla,** which is surrounded by a layer called the **cortex.** The outermost layer is the **cuticle.** Even though the hair shaft itself is constructed of non-living protein, changes to the surface of the cuticle can influence the appearance of the hair. The surface of the cuticle is arranged in a pattern resembling fish scales, and if the pattern is disrupted, the hair will appear dull. When the surface is undisturbed, the hair appears shiny. When permanent dyes are used to color the hair, they stain the cortex layer. To reach the cortex, the dye passes through the cuticle and usually disrupts its surface. Conditioners and cream rinses help to restore the cuticle.

Like the skin, the hair shaft is no longer living, although new cells are regenerated by the hair bulb, embedded in the dermis near the hair papilla. Natural hair color is influenced by the presence of melanin and other pigments. Melanin occurs in a range of colors and concentrations. It is produced in the hair papilla and is under both genetic and environmental control. Aging results in a decline in melanin production in the hair papilla. Lacking melanin, hair strands turn white.

Identify the location and function of the following structures on Figures 16-2 and in the hair follicle slide under the microscope.

arrector pili muscle

hair bulb

hair papilla

hair shaft

sebaceous gland

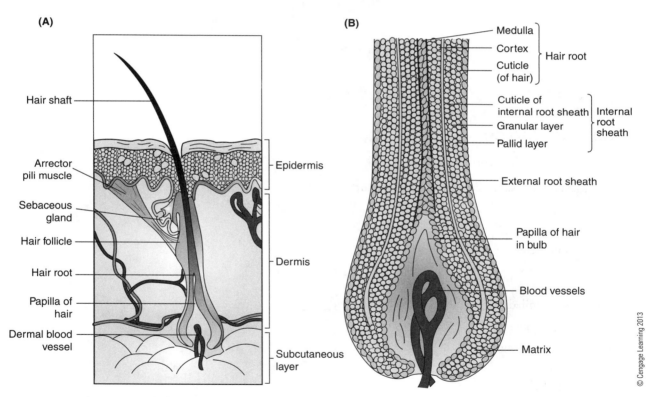

FIGURE 16-2: A. The structure of a hair within its follicle. B. The follicle expands at its base to form the bulb, which contains the dermal papilla.

NAILS

The purpose of the fingernails is to protect and stabilize the fingertips. Like hair follicles and outer layers of the skin, the fingernails are made up of non-living keratin. New growth originates from the nail root, which extends under the skin surface. The part of the nail that extends past the skin is the hyponychium.

© Cengage Learning 2013

Identify the location and function of the following structures on Figures 16-3.

hyponychium

nail body

nail root

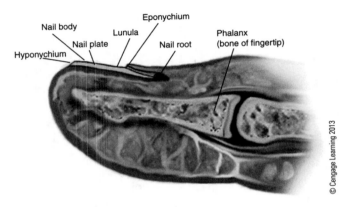

FIGURE 16-3: Structures of the fingernail.

LABORATORY REPORT QUESTIONS

Multiple Choice

Circle the letter of the correct answer.

1. The layer of the skin that is exposed at the surface is the _____.

    a. epidermis
    b. dermis
    c. subcutaneous layer
    d. hypodermis

2. The highly coiled glands in the dermis are the _____.

    a. sebaceous glands
    b. arrector pili muscles
    c. sweat glands
    d. hair follicles

3. The living portion of human hair is the _____.

    a. medulla
    b. cuticle
    c. bulb
    d. shaft

4. What is the function of the fingernails?

   a. mineral balance

   b. stabilize the fingertips

   c. protect from UV radiation

   d. cool the skin

5. What is the function of melanocytes?

   a. mineral balance

   b. stabilize the fingertips

   c. protect from UV radiation

   d. cool the skin

Matching

Match the phrases in Column A with the structures in Column B.

Column A

_____ 1. Secretes oils onto the hair follicle

_____ 2. Inner portion of the hair follicle

_____ 3. Contains blood vessels and nerves

_____ 4. Causes the hairs to stand up

_____ 5. Outer surface of the hair follicle

Column B

a. cuticle

b. dermis

c. sebaceous gland

d. medulla

e. arrector pili muscle

Long Answer

1. What role does adipose tissue play in the hypodermis?

2. Why is individual appearance important in humans?

3. How does the skin cope with abrasion and exposure to injury?

4. How are skin, hair, and nails similar to each other? How are they different?

5. What is the role of melanocytes in the skin?

COSMETICS LAB

At the completion of this exercise, the student should be able to:

- Identify the types of cosmetics in use
- Explain why people use cosmetics
- Identify the functions of the common chemicals found in cosmetics

MATERIALS

Ingredients listed for each cosmetic

INTRODUCTION

Cosmetics and body art have existed throughout much of human history. The remains of ice mummies from areas as isolated from each other as Siberia, the Alps, and Peru show intricate tattoos. The ancient Egyptians were buried with their perfumes and cosmetics. Body art has served a number of functions throughout history. Humans use it to advertise their personal status—economic, social, and marital. In pre-revolutionary France, pale, untanned skin indicated wealth and power. Only the rich could avoid the manual labor that produced tanned skin—something that was considered a disfigurement. In many tribal societies in Africa, scar patterns indicate clan association and adult status. In the South Pacific, tattoos demonstrate familial relationships. At one time in the Middle East, unmarried but available women stained their feet red with henna to announce they were looking for marriage offers. As Western cultures have become increasingly youth focused, cosmetics are used increasingly to camouflage or deemphasize wrinkles and other signs of age.

Body art can be categorized as permanent, semi-permanent, and temporary. Permanent art includes tattoos, piercing, and scarification and usually lasts throughout one's lifetime. Semi-permanent art lasts several days to months. Examples of semi-permanent body art include the dying of hair and the use of pigments like henna or woad on the skin. Once the hair grows out, the dyed color is gone. Similarly, henna or woad penetrate only the epidermal layers of the skin. As the skin is shed, the colors fade. Temporary body art is usually applied and removed within a 24-hour period. Examples include the use of eye shadow and lipstick.

Cosmetics and perfumes have been used throughout history to camouflage and prevent disease. Woad—the blue pigment used by the Celts and Picts—is both astringent (preventing bleeding) and antibacterial (preventing infection). Warriors decorated themselves with woad before battle to protect themselves as well as intimidate their enemies. Similarly during prehistoric times, henna was used for decoration in Yemen and Morocco. The kohl used to decorate the eyes in ancient Egypt contains a form of lead that is relatively harmless to humans but lethal to common parasites that infect the eyes. Used for their scent, lavender, patchouli, and sandalwood also have medicinal properties—the basis behind aromatherapy. Lavender and thyme have both been shown to kill MRSA (methicillin-resistant Staphylococcus aureus) when applied to the infected skin, as either an oil or a decoction (mashing the leaves and stems and then boiling them).

WHAT ARE COSMETICS?

Temporary make-up consists of several common materials. While the formulas have changed over the centuries, the basic components have remained the same. Pigments provide color and coverage. Titanium, iron, and zinc oxides, talc, kaolin clay, and coal tar-based colors are used as pigments. Current law prohibits the use of any organic pigments in eye make-up. Carriers are necessary to spread the pigment over the skin. The most common carriers are oils and waxes. These hold the pigments in place and also act as emollients to soften the skin. Fragrances are often added to cover the odor as bacteria digest the carrier oils. Modern cosmetics usually contain antioxidants and preservatives to prevent bacterial growth and decomposition of the oils and pigments. Glycerin, sugars, or propylene glycol are added to act as humectants, drawing moisture into the skin.

Prior to the early 1900s, most people made their own cosmetics or purchased cosmetics that were handmade in small batches. Today, almost all cosmetics are commercially prepared. Many people are surprised to learn they can make some of the cosmetics they currently purchase. This lab exercise provides an opportunity to make some simple cosmetics.

COSMETIC FORMULAS

Lip Balm

This simple lip balm contains no pigments. If you want to include flavoring, be careful to use only consumable oils. Some oils, like cinnamon and clove, are highly concentrated and may irritate the lips. Many pharmacies carry small bottles of candy flavorings that can be used as an alternative to concentrated flavor oils. Warning: If you are allergic to bees or bee stings, do not use this product.

15 mL melted beeswax
30 mL coconut oil
1 mL honey
2 drops flavoring of choice (oil-based)

Heat beeswax, coconut oil, and honey until melted.

Remove from heat and stir in flavoring.

Pour mixture into a small jar or tube.

If you prefer to use herbs or citrus peels as flavoring, add to the oil and wax as they melt. Strain before packaging.

Lavender Hand and Heel Cream

This thick cream is especially effective at soothing dry, cracked skin. Lavender has antibacterial and antifungal properties and has been used for centuries to soothe and heal the skin. For greatest effectiveness, apply immediately after bathing to trap the moisture in the skin.

20 mL grapeseed oil
20 mL coconut oil
5 g beeswax
5 mL vegetable glycerin
6 drops lavender oil

Over low heat, melt grapeseed and coconut oil with wax.

Remove from heat; add glycerin drop by drop while stirring.

Stir in lavender oil.

Continue stirring until thick.

Store in a sealed jar.

Foundation/Grease Paint

Foundation is basically just a pigment in oil. Theatrical make-up or a simple foundation can be made by combining an opaque pigment with an oil. Cornstarch gives a white base and can be tinted by adding paste food coloring (not the liquid in a squeeze bottle). While too heavy when compared with modern foundations, this foundation does work well for face painting and costumes and washes off with soap and water.

> 1 part coconut oil
> 1 part cornstarch
> pigment (optional)

> *Melt oil.*
> *Gently add cornstarch.*
> *Stir to combine.*
> *If desired, tint with pigment to produce desired shade.*

Sunburn Soother

While not designed to change appearances, this soothing lotion tones down the discomfort of a mild sunburn. Mint contains menthol, which evaporates and produces a cooling sensation.

> 1 cucumber
> 1 handful mint leaves
> 120 mL water
> 2 drops lavender oil

> *Peel and seed cucumber.*
> *Blend cucumber, mint leaves, and water in a blender until smooth.*
> *Strain liquid to remove any remaining solids.*
> *Add lavender oil.*
> *Store in the refrigerator.*
> *Apply to overexposed skin to soothe and cool.*

Body Butter

Sesame oil acts as a sunscreen, providing some protection from sun damage. Coconut and cocoa butter are rich in minerals, fat-soluble vitamins, and fatty acids. Rose water soothes damaged skin and provides a pleasant scent.

> 20 mL melted beeswax
> 5 mL rose water
> 120 mL cocoa butter
> 45 mL sesame oil
> 30 mL coconut oil
> 15 mL olive oil

> *Over low heat, combine wax and rose water and heat until wax is melted.*
> *Add cocoa butter and blend well.*

Remove from heat.

Combine the other oils and gradually add to the melted mixture, stirring constantly until it begins to thicken.

Pour into a glass jar. The lotion will continue to thicken as it cools.

LAB REPORT

1. Choosing two cosmetics you have at home, list each ingredient from the label and describe what each does.

2. How do the cosmetics you prepared compare with commercial products you are familiar with?

3. If you use cosmetics, why?

LABORATORY REPORT QUESTIONS

Multiple Choice

Circle the letter of the correct answer.

1. A chemical added to a cosmetic to help spread the pigment across the skin is the _____

   a. antioxidant
   b. humectant
   c. carrier
   d. dye

2. Glycerin helps to _____.

   a. draw moisture into the skin
   b. protect against sun damage
   c. add a minty flavor
   d. keep the oils from going rancid

3. Body art that extends into the dermis layers of the skin is _____.

   a. temporary
   b. semipermanent
   c. permanent
   d. no longer used

4. Titanium dioxide is used as a _____ in cosmetics.

   a. humectant
   b. carrier
   c. fragrance
   d. pigment

5. Cosmetics that lack _____ may become rancid.

   a. pigments
   b. carriers
   c. preservatives
   d. humectants

Matching

Match the description in Column A with the term in Column B.

Column A	Column B
___ 1. Blue pigment that slows both infection and bleeding	a. kohl
___ 2. Ancient Egyptian cosmetic used to protect the eyes	b. sesame oil
___ 3. Oil used as a natural sunscreen	c. lavender
___ 4. Provides a cooling note to lotions and creams	d. woad
___ 5. Fragrant oil shown to be effective in killing antibiotic-resistant bacteria	e. mint

Long Answer

1. Many cosmetics formulas contain beeswax and coconut oil. Why?

2. How can cosmetics serve a social function?

3. What role do chemicals like zinc oxide and kaolin play in cosmetics?

4. What are the benefits of cosmetics?

5. Why do many cosmetics contain humectants?

NOTES

NOTES

NOTES

NOTES